The International Library of Psychology

THE PSYCHOLOGY OF CHILDREN'S DRAWINGS

Founded by C. K. Ogden

The International Library of Psychology

DEVELOPMENTAL PSYCHOLOGY
In 32 Volumes

THE PSYCHOLOGY OF CHILDREN'S DRAWINGS

From the First Stroke to the Coloured Drawing

HELGA ENG

First published in 1931 by
Routledge

Reprinted in 1999, 2001 by
Routledge
2 Park Square, Milton Park, Abingdon, Oxfordshire OX14 4RN
711 Third Avenue, New York, NY 10017

Transferred to Digital Printing 2007

First issued in paperback 2014

Routledge is an imprint of the Taylor and Francis Group, an informa business

British Library Cataloguing in Publication Data
A CIP catalogue record for this book
is available from the British Library

The Psychology of Children's Drawings
ISBN 978-0-415-20987-8 (hbk)
ISBN 978-0-415-86440-4 (pbk)
Developmental Psychology: 32 Volumes
ISBN 978-0-415-21128-4
The International Library of Psychology: 204 Volumes
ISBN 978-0-415-19132-6

CONTENTS

PREFACE

THIS book has been written because I was provided with rich and complete material as the result of daily observation of my little niece. Her drawing from the first to the eighth year is unusually elaborate. It includes formalized, naturalistic and perspective drawings, letters, attempts at illustration, ornament, etc., and is always typically childlike and always spontaneous. She started drawing at ten months ; scribbled industriously for more than half a year, and passed through clearly defined phases. Krötzsch grasped the significance of scribbling as the fundamental process and the sign of decadence ; I find that it plays a great part in the development of the normal and healthy child's drawing up to its eighth year.

In order to make full use of the material, I have given the development of the drawing of my little niece in the first part of the book in chronological order, while in the second part I have interpreted psychologically the whole of the drawings and observations. In the first part, however, some psychological remarks have been made where they have been necessary ; in the second part, the child's expression of itself in drawing has been discussed in its relation to scribbling, schema, automatism, orientation, proportions, movement, perspective, colour, and ornament, and also with reference to development in point of time.

In the psychological analysis of my material I have made use of results of earlier investigations in this field, and have discussed the views of the authors, and in part criticized them. I mention particularly the works of W. Stern, Kerschensteiner, Levinstein, Rouma, Luquet,

Scupin, Dix, Krötzsch, and also the excellent chapter on drawing in Bühler's *The Mental Development of the Child*. I have everywhere given references. ,

In the third part, the drawing of the child is considered as an expression of its mental development, taking into account my own earlier results on the mental life of children.

In the last part I think I have been able, on the basis of my exact observations of the first beginnings of drawing, to give new proofs of the agreement between the development of children's drawings and that of the oldest folk-art.

The object of this work as a whole is to deepen and widen our knowledge of the psychology of drawing and of the child.

I owe my thanks to the Jubilee Fund of the University of Oslo for a contribution enabling me to carry out and publish the work.

HELGA ENG.

OSLO.

PREFACE TO THE SECOND EDITION

THE present edition is mainly a reprint of the first edition. Part of the chapter " Children's Drawings as an Expression of Their Mental Development " and a few shorter sections have been rewritten, and a number of minor alterations and corrections have been made.

The words ' formula ' and ' formal ' are used throughout the text, as in the first edition, instead of the now accepted ' schema ' and ' schematic ', but my readers will be able to transpose the one set of words for the other. I also prefer the terms ' swing scribbling ' and ' round scribbling ' to ' wavy scribbling ' and ' circular scribbling '.

HELGA ENG.

OSLO.
October, 1953

THE PSYCHOLOGY
OF CHILDREN'S DRAWINGS

THE DRAWING OF A CHILD FROM THE FIRST STROKE TO COLOURED DRAWINGS MADE AT EIGHT YEARS OF AGE

SINCE the Italian historian C. Ricci [1] published, in the year 1887, his famous pamphlet on the art of children, a number of works have appeared which have made known to us the main characteristics of the free drawings of children. In order to enlarge and deepen this knowledge, particularly in the psychological direction, it is necessary, as many psychologists have pointed out, to make exact and complete observations of the development of the drawings of a single child. The following study is a contribution in this direction and concerns the drawing of a child from the first to the eighth year.

I was able to observe the drawing of my little niece Margaret from the first stroke to the comparatively complicated compositions of her seventh to eighth year, and collect examples of it. Her early bodily and mental development had nothing unusual about it ; she learnt to walk and talk, as most children do, at the age of one. She had no brothers or sisters, and was not influenced in her drawing by playmates, a fact which was particularly favourable for the study of her. Luquet, who followed the drawing of his eldest daughter Simonne with great profit, found the results of the observation of her younger brother, whose spontaneous drawing was continually

[1] Corrado Ricci, *L'arte dei bambini.* German Translation, C. Ricci, *Kinderkunst,* Leipzig, 1906.

influenced by the example, criticism, and advice of his sister, much more scanty.[1] Margaret had no instruction in drawing, but every now and then a drawing was made in front of her, in the first two and three years quite frequently, later on seldom, in the last years, almost never. This was usually done only at her own wish, and the drawing generally represented an object which she had chosen. Nobody asked her to draw, or kept her at it, nor were her drawings corrected and her mistakes pointed out. Nor did anyone ask her about her drawings ; if in this respect exceptions occurred the fact will be mentioned later. All that was done was to see that pencil and paper were always present whenever she wanted to draw ; when she was drawing she was observed, and all her spontaneous remarks, in fact everything that had in any way to do with the drawing, were written down. Usually she chattered while she was drawing and explained her artistic products, nevertheless she had no notion that observations were being made of her activities, until she discovered, when she was over six years old, that I was collecting her drawings. This discovery may have somewhat stimulated her interest in drawing in the latter part of the time. She had plenty of opportunity for looking at pictures and picture-books, and her surroundings were always such as to incite her to pictorial representations, but the reception and digestion of her impressions in this respect were entirely spontaneous, without any direct influence on the part of her family.

In the first three years I also observed the development of her speech.

Only a part of the drawings which were collected and preserved during the course of the years will be discussed and reproduced here. In making my choice I kept in mind the object of giving, by means of examples of each noteworthy step in progress, a complete view of the development of her drawing.

[1] G. H. Luquet, *Les dessins d'un enfant*, xv, xvi.

FIRST AND SECOND YEAR

Margaret made her first stroke before she began to speak, at the age of ten months. I drew for her a little girl, which she looked at attentively ; the pencil was put in her hand and she put it on the paper and made two small lines, which she looked at with much interest (Fig. 1).

The experiment was not repeated for some time, and there is no further progress to record until she was a year and some months old.

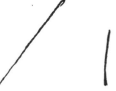

FIG. 1.—THE FIRST
STROKE. 0 ; 10. 1/1.

At 1 ; 2, 2 (at the age of one year, two months, and two days— I shall make use of this way of giving the age in what follows), she drew a few uncertain strokes, which appear to exhibit typical wavy scribbling, the usual result of the first attempts of a child to draw (Fig. 2). A week later (1 ; 2, 8), she produced strong and

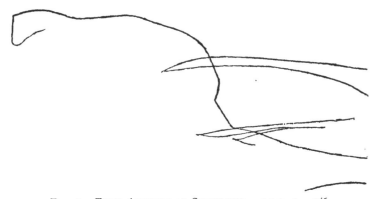

FIG. 2.—FIRST ATTEMPT AT SCRIBBLING. 1 ; 2, 2. 5/6.

clear wavy scribbling in the following way : she moved her hand quickly outwards and described a slightly curved line, then reversed and drew a curved line inwards, in the opposite direction, and so on. At the turning-point the line is often pointed, but generally somewhat rounded, now and then making a loop. Each new line is usually drawn under the previous one, but often over it, or irregularly. Wavy scribbling is, in the first period, the fundamental form of a child's drawing, although not exclusively produced. Shorter strokes, points, angles, bent lines, also often occur. On the other hand, we never meet with circles, zig-zag lines, spirals and so on. Wavy scribbling has nothing to do with intelligible representation, and does not express the child's ideas, but it naturally contributes to the child's practice in understanding and drawing lines, by training eye and hand.

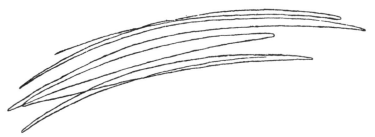

FIG. 3.—WAVY SCRIBBLING. FRAGMENT. 1 ; 4, 10. ABOUT 1/2.

At first Margaret often took hold of the pencil the wrong way round, but from the age of 1 ; 2, 9, she generally managed to hold it correctly. At the beginning she sometimes used the right and sometimes the left hand, but from the age of 1 ; 4, 10, she drew only with the right hand, although she was not told to do so. Wavy scribbling continued for about four months until 1 ; 6, without any further visible improvement apart from the line becoming firmer and surer. A typical example of well-developed wavy scribbling is given in Fig. 3 (1 ; 4, 10). It was usually placed on the paper as a dense compact mass.

Major and Dix have also observed that wavy scribbling is the first step in the drawing of children. The first drawings of Major's son, at 1 ; 0, 1 ; 1, 1 ; 2, 1 ; 4,

1 ; 6, have exactly the same character as the drawings of Margaret at about the same age.[1] Dix also, whose son Walther-Heinz began to draw at the age of 11 months, mentions wavy scribbling.[2] Krötzsch gives an example of wavy scribbling at 1 ; 7.[3]

· At 1 ; 6, Margaret changed to circular scribbling (Fig. 4). The change took place fairly suddenly. At 1 ; 6, 15, she scribbled in well-defined circles, while in the days just preceding this she had produced unusually clear and pure wavy scribbling. The change may be the result of imitation. Her father had drawn for her on that day about a dozen different objects, among which were several rounded figures such as a watch, a ball, wheel, and so on. Round and oval scribbling in dense masses in the middle of the paper characterized her drawing for the following couple of months.

At 1 ; 8, she commenced a new phase which may be called variegated scribbling (Fig. 5). Along with circular and wavy scribbling we now have straight lines, angles, crosses, zig-zag lines and loops, forming altogether a tangle of lines. About the same time, a new development appears, viz., from scribbling in masses to scattered scribbling. In the following period the lines are loosened up as it were, and are put on paper more widely separated from one another. At 1 ; 8, 18, her scribbling was put for the first time on to the surface of the paper in little groups, and thenceforth the various forms and lines were more consciously drawn, and repeated.

About three weeks later a further step forward was made ; a meaning was given to the scribbling. At 1 ; 9, 10, Margaret drew a few lines crossing one another, and said : " flag ", " flower ", " dress ", " apron ", " wall ". She thus connected for the first time an idea with what she had drawn.

[1] D. Major, *First Steps in Mental Growth*, pp. 46 et seq.
[2] K. W. Dix, *Körperliche und geistige Entwicklung eines Kindes*, pp. 69, 70.
[3] W. Krötzsch, *Rhythmus und Form in der freien Kinderzeichnung*, pp. 5 et seq.

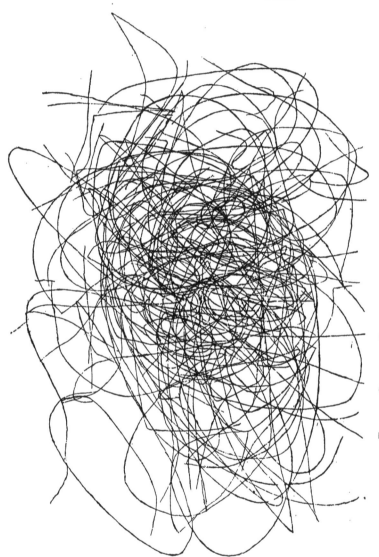

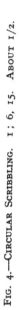

FIG. 4.—CIRCULAR SCRIBBLING. 1 ; 6, 15. ABOUT 1/2.

A few days later, 1 ; 9, 13, as she was engaged in scribbling, she said : " draw Mama ". She drew a few small zig-zag lines which ended in a longer line and said :

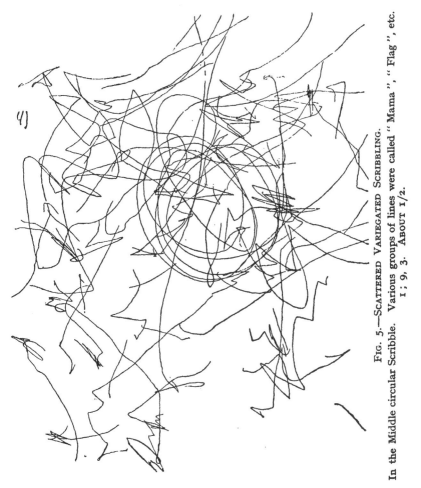

FIG. 5.—SCATTERED VARIEGATED SCRIBBLING. Various groups of lines were called " Mama ", " Flag ", etc. 1 ; 9, 3. ABOUT 1/2. In the Middle circular Scribble.

" that's Mama ", then she said : " draw flag "—made a straight line—" that's flag ". She continued : " draw dress "—a few·lines scribbled together. In the same way she drew the floor, a cock-a-doodle-doo, a mirror, and so on. She thus announced beforehand what she was going to draw. She generally produced a small dense zig-zag scribble ending in a longer line (Fig. 6), the whole forming a connected mass of lines running all over the paper. Ekki Krötzsch called a similar figure a man at 2 ; 1.[1]

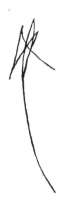

FIG. 6.—"MAMA." 1 ; 9, 13.   1/1.

Margaret thus came quite on her own initiative to use her drawing as a means of expression. We had already noticed six months previously that she understood the meaning of pictures and drawings ; at 1 ; 4, 8 she spoke her own name when she noticed the child on a picture of the Madonna, and described a picture of a dog as a " bow-wow ". She was probably able to understand pictures and drawings earlier than that. This confirms what has been observed in other parts of a child's mental development, that the receptive side of an activity is developed earlier than the productive.

A few weeks later, at 1 ; 9, 22, she made a further step forward in separating Mama and bow-wow, each drawn as a clear and simple group of lines ; both drawings have the same form and consist of two curves linked together, finishing in a hook directed upwards (Fig. 7). At the same time she began to make a figure, which was predominant for about a week ; a single curve, sometimes open, but often closed by beginning and end running across or parallel to one another. A straight line was often added to the curve, generally running downwards or to the right. She also practised

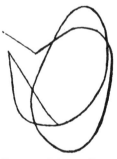

FIG. 7.—"MAMA." 1 ; 9, 22.   1/2.

[1] Krötzsch, loc. cit., p. 9.

straight lines, longer and shorter. Sometimes the whole exercise consisted only in a long line ending in a round loop (Fig. 8).

As it then appeared, this drawing, clearly to be distinguished from scribbling, was the forerunner of her first formula drawing.[1]

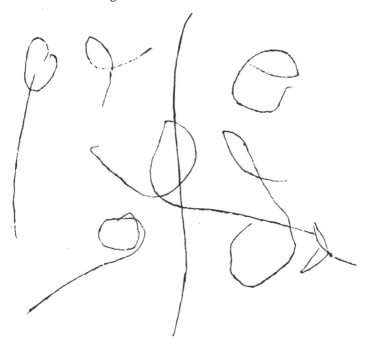

FIG. 8.—ISOLATED SCRIBBLING. 1 ; 9, 26. ABOUT 10/11.

It is a fact that children who draw, attack first of all the problem—the touchstone and goal of all art—of drawing the human form. Margaret was no exception. The first drawing with which she entered the formula period, was supposed to represent " Mama ". This is a round figure and two straight lines, which are often vertical, but also frequently sloping downwards or quite horizontal, as in Fig. 9 (1 ; 10). This figure is now

[1] See Footnote, p. 109 (*Trans.*).

repeated endlessly with ease and clarity. But it does not only stand for Mama, but sometimes also for a flower or a flag. She is no doubt thinking of a flower with its stalk or a flag on its pole, particularly when, as often happens, she only makes one line instead of two. At any rate, in the case of Mama the figure is a genuine formula drawing, the same which according to Ricci

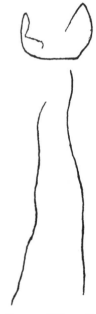

occurs in 99 out of a 100 cases when the child is first pleased with the idea of drawing something. It is a circle or a square with two vertical lines. "What, a head and legs all alone?—certainly, that is enough for seeing, eating and walking." [1] Margaret's formula man would, however, have had to confine himself to the last activity alone, for eyes and mouth are missing, and the head only consists of an empty circle. German child psychologists have described this primitive man, consisting only of head and legs, as *Kopffüssler*, and the French have called it *têtard*. Margaret reached the formalized stage unusually early, at 1 ; 10. Stern's son, who took an extraordinary interest in drawing and showed a gift unusual for his age, made his first formalized drawing, a picture

FIG. 9.—"MAMA."
1 ; 10. 1/1.

of his sister, at the age of 3 ; 2½. It almost appears little more than a scribble, for head and trunk run together as a circular scribble; arms and legs, however, can be clearly distinguished.[2]

Major's son produced his first drawing, which was more than a scribble, at 2 ; 6, 21 ; on this day he imitated intentionally and successfully an O which had often been

[1] Ricci, *Kinderkunst*, pp. 11 and 12.
[2] W. Stern, "Die zeichnerische Entwicklung eines Knaben ", *Z. angew. Ps.*, 3, p. 5.

drawn for him as an example. But only in the age of three years did he draw his first formalized man,[1] although from the end of his first year he always received a certain amount of instruction in drawing. Continual efforts were made, by showing him how to draw, to get him to imitate what was done. According to the Scupins' report of their child, his first clear outline drawing, at the age of 2 ; 9, 2, was the " moon face ", because this was most often drawn for him as an example, accompanied by the verse " dot, dot, comma, dash, there's the moon-face ". His mother had to draw it for him innumerable times, and as soon as the drawing was finished on the slate he rubbed it out again eagerly, in order to see it made once more. At the age of 2 ; 4, 11, he asked for this drawing exactly sixty times, without showing the slightest signs of tiring of this infinitely monotonous game. He followed exactly the repetition of the verse, and if it were once forgotten, he rubbed out the drawing angrily, even while it was being made, as valueless.[2] At the age of 2 ; 9, 7, he drew his first real formalized drawing, " Mama " : a circle with two vertical lines, just like that of Margaret ; but on being asked, he was able to complete it with eyes, nose, mouth, and ears, hair consisting of five strokes, and even with shoes.[3] As we see from this, the primitive formula of a child is not always so imperfect because it is not able to draw, but also because the child is not sufficiently advanced in spontaneous conception and drawing.

In the case of Walther-Heinz Dix, the first conscious drawing he made was also the " moon face " so often drawn for him (1 ; 8). It consisted only of an open circle with some lines in the middle, not much more than a circular scribble ; it was not until 2 ; 2 that he drew it as a formula, with a nose and two circles as eyes. He accompanied the drawing with the little verse in a somewhat shortened form, " dot, dot, comma, dash, moon ". At 2 ; 3, he produced a picture of his best-beloved object,

[1] Major, loc. cit., pp. 55 et seq.
[2] Ernst und Gertrud Scupin, Bubis erste Kindheit, pp. 130, 165.
[3] loc cit., p. 170.

a locomotive, for the drawing of which he never tired of asking. In this he showed real genius in making use of the technique which he had mastered in scribbling. The boiler of the locomotive was a long narrow strip of shading lines, consisting of almost straight wavy lines, the wheels were two circles, the chimney a straight line, the smoke a simple spiral scribble.[1] Ekki Krötzsch drew his first formalized human being at 2 ; 4, but as in the case of Margaret he did not retain it, but lost it again.[2] The first formalized drawing made by little Simonne Luquet was produced at 3 ; 4, 13.[3]

After Margaret had thus set up a record in the matter of early formalized drawing, a reaction appears to have supervened ; at any rate, she spent the following three weeks in scribbling. Nevertheless this had a different character from the earlier product of the kind, and appeared almost like intentional practice. The formula of a circle and a line was repeated as a scribble, without her attaching any particular meaning to it ; she practised circles and spirals, and several times made a strong circular scribble in a dense mass in the middle of the paper. The most characteristic feature of this time, however, was the practising of rectangles, to an extent which might almost be described as systematic. For some weeks she continually drew long and almost straight lines, continuing with a sharp or somewhat rounded bend, and with the next stroke almost at right angles to the first. At 1 ; 10, 5, she really succeeded in drawing an angle of exactly 90° formed of two almost straight lines (Fig. 10). As a rule, however, only open angles were made, but it sometimes looked as if she were trying to turn these into a quadrilateral by cross strokes. At the same period, 1 ; 10, 5, she made her first picture of her-self : a circle with many strokes for legs ; in the circle there are four or five marks consisting of small scribbled zig-zag lines, probably the eyes (Fig. 10).

[1] Dix, *loc. cit.*, pp. 71 *et seq.*   [2] Krötzsch, *loc. cit.*, pp. 13, 69 *et seq.*
[3] Luquet, *loc. cit.*, pp. 3, 23, 122 ; Plates 1, 38, 39.

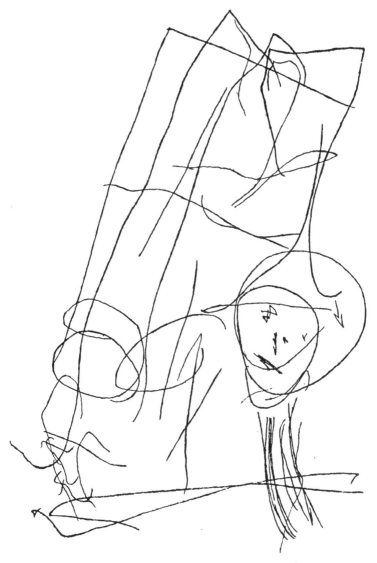

FIG. 10.—TOP LEFT, SCRIBBLING AS PRACTICE FOR FLAG. BOTTOM
RIGHT, MARGARET. 1 ; 10, 5. ABOUT 2/5.

Krötzsch remarks, that the point produced by the child when it has reached this stage consists of circular scribble : " For the child it is in reality a spiral compressed into the smallest space possible." [1]

This is certainly a correct observation ; when children in the lowest classes at school are told to dot their i's, the dots are usually made from spirals compressed into the smallest possible space. Margaret's drawings show that the point also results from other forms of elementary scribbling, viz., also from zig-zag lines compressed together. Margaret, by the way, had produced points even at the beginning of her scribbling period in another way, by a short contact of the pencil with the paper. The point in this case resulted from the straight lines which in wavy scribbling appear together with the bent line. For she often drew first a long line, then lifted the pencil for a moment, and then again touched the paper for a moment, in order to produce a point in the continuation of the line ; the result has the form of a note of exclamation, the line of which is very much prolonged (Fig. 11).

At 1 ; 10, 14, she produced a four-cornered figure with two corners round and one rather pointed (Fig. 12) ; as appears from my notes, she drew on the next day an almost regular, elongated rectangle, of which only one corner was somewhat rounded ; this drawing was unfortunately not preserved.

Several of the characteristic features of Margaret's drawing at this period may be traced to the influence of certain drawings made in front of her. At about this time, viz., from about the twenty-second month, she was shown a great deal of drawing, not to teach her, but to amuse her. Almost every day she asked to have something drawn for her, naming the object herself. She constantly and repeatedly asked for a flag and a flower. The flag was drawn with red and blue pencil and shaded, the flag-pole with an ordinary pencil. The flower was a formalized tulip, the blossom, consisting of three large

[1] Krötzsch, *loc. cit.*, p. 14.

spikes with a round lower part, was drawn in red pencil and shaded, and a straight stem with a leaf on each side was put in with blue pencil. It was exceptional for her to ask for anything else to be drawn, a little girl, a dress, the foot-stool or the sofa, the " bow-wow ", horse and cart ; she usually only repeated such requests two or three times. It is not easy to tell why she preferred the two particular drawings ; perhaps because they were the only ones made in red and blue—the colours usually preferred by children—whilst the other objects were generally drawn only with ordinary pencil. She herself began by drawing only with an ordinary pencil and did

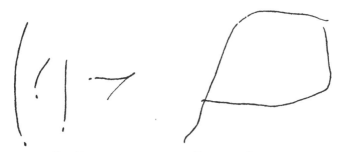

FIG. 11.—THE POINT, ARISING FROM THE LINE. FRAGMENT. 1 ; I, 11. 1/1.

FIG. 12.—QUADRILATERAL. 1 ; 10, 14. 1/2.

not commence to use red and blue pencils until her twenty-second month.

She invariably began her drawing each day with the demand for a flag to be drawn, and then watched excitedly how the flag was produced. As soon as the drawing was finished, she asked for it again. This was repeated three to five times. The flower, which usually took second place, had also to be repeated as a rule two or three times, sometimes as many as five. This confirms what has been observed by many child psychologists, viz., that the pleasure of the child in its own drawing and in the drawing of others, consists mainly in its interest in the movement, in the action. But the interest of seeing things pictured also plays a large part. This is shown by the fact that Margaret at this time not only took a lively interest in the process of the flag being drawn, but also had a special preference for the Norwegian flag, both the object itself and pictures of it. At 1 ; 11, she saw, for example, the picture of some children with flags in their hands, whereupon she said with great interest and very excitedly, "that's flag" and repeated this several times with great joy.

Dix tells us about Walther-Heinz that he also showed at times a strong preference for certain objects which had then to be drawn for him again and again. Among these, the locomotive was pre-eminent, for he had in

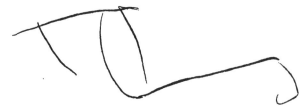

FIG. 13.—FLAG. RED PENCIL. 1 ; 10, 24. 1/2.

every way a strong preference for it, both for the real thing, as well as for the toy, in stories and so on.[1]

At 1 ; 10, 24, after her innumerable practices with straight lines, angles, and rectangles, Margaret for the first time announced her intention of drawing a flag. The result was a lop-sided rectangle with the fourth side missing ; a long stroke, no doubt intended to close it, was made too far to one side (Fig. 13). On the next day she drew a few rectangles which were not very successful ; they show, it is true, the elongated form of the flag, but are askew and have several open corners. In addition, she drew a circular scribble with a stem. At 1 ; 11, she succeeded two or three times quite well in drawing a tulip in the form of a zig-zag line and a rounded end

[1] Dix, loc. cit., pp. 74, 93.

(Fig. 14) ; she also produced a flag-shaped figure and some other scribble. At 1 ; 11, 21, she remarked concerning a bell-shaped figure hanging from a boldly curved stem (the whole being probably rather an accidental product) : " that's flower ". She was satisfied for the time with these attempts to draw a flower and a flag. Spring came ; she was more out of doors, and in the summer months drawing was almost given up. When she took it up again in the autumn, her interest for other models had grown.

Margaret's apparently methodical practice, and her attempts to draw flags and flowers, cannot be compared with the attempt of the school child to draw from a copy

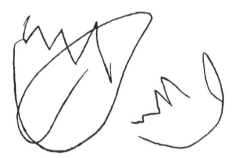

FIG. 14.—FLOWER. RED AND BLUE PENCIL. 1 ; 11. 1/2.

or a model. Margaret neither looked at my drawings nor compared them with her own ; as a rule she had no purpose in making the latter, but drew and scribbled just as it occurred to her, although she certainly must have had an object when she said expressly " draw flag ". The fact that the usual result was the two forms flag and flower, or parts of them, may have been due to these having been so firmly retained in her memory by practice, that they flowed, as it were, from her hand when she made her attempts at drawing. Nevertheless, the reproduction is unclear and incomplete, which was partly to be accounted for by the imperfect correlation between movement and imagination, and partly also by

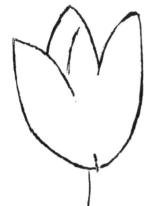

the fact that a child's grasp of things is unclear and incomplete, and its memory picture the same. That this is actually the case is amply proved by Margaret's later attempts to draw a flag, when over six years old.[1]

At about 1 ; 10, and subsequently, she often asked me, when I had finished the flag, to be allowed to draw the flag-pole. Her flag-pole was generally more or less bent and not always placed accurately on the edge of the flag. It appeared that she was capable of self-criticism, for after one, or generally several attempts, she finally asked me to draw the flag-pole myself. She also drew the stem, when I had finished the flower, and generally placed it quite correctly under the flower; although it also was often more or less crooked, she sometimes succeeded in a very good stroke. Indeed, at 1 ; 10, 17, she astonished us by a quite surprising success, producing a stem twelve centimetres long, which nowhere departed noticeably from a straight line (Fig. 15).

Ruskin tells us that, according to his observation, a great artist can draw any line excepting a straight line. One of

FIG. 15.—
STRAIGHT LINE,
DRAWN AS STEM
OF A FLOWER.
1 ; 10, 17. 1/2.

[1] Cf. p. 74.

his pupils, E. Cooke, who is known by his reform of the teaching of drawing, quotes Ruskin's words and criticizes the teaching of his time. The teaching of drawing, he says, commences with straight lines, angles and geometrical figures, which mean nothing to the child, who cannot construct from them any of the living creatures which interest it ; the child prefers life and movement, and would like to draw human beings, horses, houses, and ships. While Nature, he tells us, has fitted the child for play and for art, the school demands geometry ; when it wishes to draw many lines, it is confined to one; when it wishes to draw something whole, it is forced to represent single parts. Neither the child nor primitive man begins with a geometrical line ; the history of graphic art is hidden in a scribble.[1] Many other writers have also attacked geometrical drawing, which takes all life and all action out of the child's drawing, by making the lines straight.

The dominance of geometrical drawing in schools is no doubt mainly due to the influence of Pestalozzi. He started with the straight line, the lines were joined to angles, and the angles made into four-sided figures. Pestalozzi regarded the four-sided figure as the simplest form, the fundamental form, and built up on this basis his teaching concerning drawing and form. Herbart supposed the triangle to be the easiest fundamental form, while Fröbel took the sphere as the perfect form, at once the simplest and most complex, hence the fundamental form in all teaching.

Fröbel came nearest to the truth. The first form which develops from the tangle of scribble, is, as we saw, a more or less incomplete circle ; it is the first structure that the child draws on its own initiative. There is therefore good psychological reason for the sharp attacks made by modern teachers of drawing upon the limitation to straight-lined, rectangular drawing usual in elementary instruction. But, perhaps, they go too far when they

---

[1] E. T. Cooke, *The ABC of Drawing*, pp. 145 *et seq.*

wish to banish the straight line and the rectangle completely from children's drawing.   Margaret practised on
her own initiative straight lines, angles, and rectangles
from the age of two ; and Walther-Heinz was already
drawing, at 2 ; 3, very good rectangles as necessary parts
of his beloved locomotive.   It is true that, in these cases,
the reason is to be found in the fact that one of the
children preferred a flag and the other a locomotive, but
nevertheless we may draw the conclusion that this kind
of drawing is not quite unnatural, even in a child's
earliest years.

We must mention a new acquisition of Margaret's
about this time, in her drawings of human beings, viz.,
that her eyes were opened to certain details, such as hair,
eyes, fingers, and legs.   She did not, however, add these
to the formalized human being hitherto drawn by her ;
on the contrary, her attention appeared to be so strongly
attracted by them, as to suppress for the time the comparatively correct, if very primitive, idea of the human
form, which she had made her own and expressed in her
drawing.   At 1 ; 10, 20, she drew, as she had already
been doing for the last two or three weeks on occasion,
circles with points in them, and called the points eyes ;
but there were not two eyes alone, but a great many.
In the smaller circle, which no doubt represents the head,
a considerable number of " eyes " are placed ; above
this she puts some strokes and said " hair ".   To the
larger circle she then added a line sloping upwards and
said " that's a leg " : another line : " that's another
leg " (Fig. 16).   There is a curious illogicality in her
drawing, inasmuch as she puts in two legs quite correctly,
but a considerable number of eyes.   As a matter of
fact, she still had no clear conception of the number
two.   This first came to her some months later, at 2 ; 7.
Several months before the production of this drawing
she had already made use of the expression " other "
concerning her other shoe, other stocking, etc.   She thus
had a more or less clear conception of a pair of objects

belonging together, " a double " as it were, but not of the numerical concept two. And this concept of a double can be applied to the legs, but not to the eyes, probably because the expressions " other shoe ", " other stocking " were used daily in her dressing and undressing, while other expressions which could inculcate the idea of a

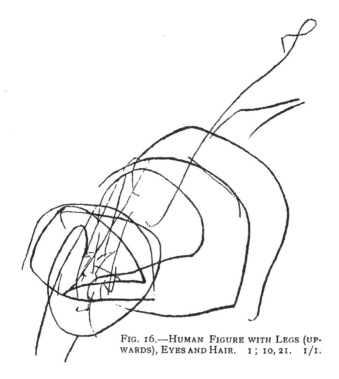

Fig. 16.—Human Figure with Legs (up-wards), Eyes and Hair. 1 ; 10, 21. 1/1.

double in relation to her eyes did not occur. This idea was connected with certain things only, and could not be applied generally.

During the whole of this time, viz., the end of the second year, she continued to scribble from time to time, mainly circular scribble, but also wavy lines, zig-zag lines, circles, and straight strokes ; partly as a dense scribble, partly as scattered scribbling or isolated exercises.

At 1 ; 11, 22, she drew for the first time " fingers ",
each in the form of a straight stroke with a three-cornered
loop at the end. They formed part of a remarkably
complete human form, consisting of a circular scribble,
the head, and four eyes, a straight line, the neck, which
passes into a fresh circular scribble, smaller than the
head and forming the body : below this the two legs
meeting at their ends, and sideways, in the middle of

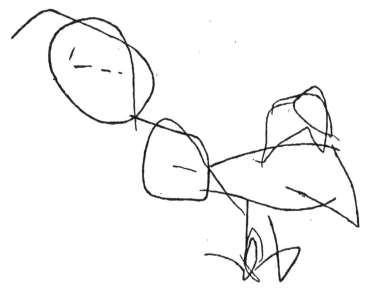

Fig. 17.—" Mama." Red Pencil. 1 ; 11, 22. About 5/6.

the legs, are the fingers, two at each side. The whole
figure is horizontal, only the head is sloping a little
upwards. This was called " Mama " (Fig. 17).

This drawing was repeated on the same and on the
next day, and developed into a new human formula, at
the age of 1 ; 11, 25. First the head appears as a circle ;
from the head a line, representing the neck, is drawn
straight downwards ; this passes into the body as a
double circular scribble. Two straight lines form the

legs, and right at the bottom a few small cross lines close together perhaps represent the feet. Eyes, hair, and fingers have again disappeared ; the two last, by the way, each only appeared once. This drawing, however, forms a fairly complete and well-proportioned human form, with head, body, and legs in fairly correct relation, and carried out with a clear firm line.

This formula was now only drawn in a vertical position. It was not, as at 1 ; 10, also used for the designation of other objects, but only as representing a human being ; " that's Mama ", " that's man " (Fig. 18). This drawing, which shows a capacity for drawing highly developed for a two-year-old child, marked the close of Margaret's second year of life and first year of drawing.

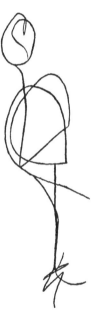

FIG. 18.—" MAMA " (OR " MAN "). 1; 11, 25. 1/2.

THE THIRD YEAR

We have seen that Margaret has advanced further in drawing in the course of her second year than is usual for a normal child. We then find that this human formula, produced at the end of the second year, and comparatively highly developed, was not retained and developed further, but degenerated into circular scribbling. At 2 ; 0, 4, she again drew " Mama "—a gigantic double circular scribble as a head, a second, only one-third as large as the head and partly covering it, as body, two strokes as legs, joined by a cross stroke ; a couple of strokes made rather casually close to the body, perhaps represent the arms. The whole is badly shaped and badly proportioned. The vertical position has also been lost again ; the figure slopes downwards to the right, as in earlier cases. To make up for this, the features are better given : " That's

Mama's eyes, nose and mouth." The nose and mouth are two long, fairly correctly placed lines; as in earlier cases, there were too many eyes, scattered about in a chance fashion. A few light strokes above them perhaps represent hair (Fig. 19).

Here we meet again the same trait we observed earlier: The details are well drawn, but the outlines are defective. Attention is directed to the details, and the outlines are

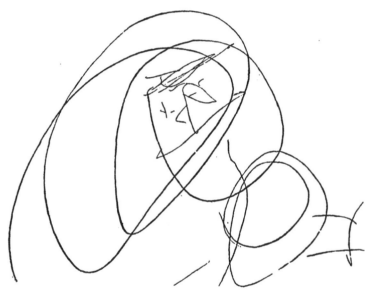

FIG. 19.—" MAMA." 2 ; 0, 4. ABOUT 1/2.

badly done. It would appear that the child's mind has not the power to get a complete view of the whole, and, at the same time, to observe the details. E. Brown observed a similar alternation between detail and general outline in a child's drawing.[1] Probably we are dealing here with a psychological law of great generality. F. Krueger finds that a real grasp of the whole tends to check the grasp of details ; vice versa, but in a less

[1] Elmer E. Brown, *Notes on Children's Drawings*, p. 71.

degree, the particular aspects of the whole are obscured by an isolated grasp of detail.[1] F. Seifert also observed in his experiments an alternate obstruction of whole and of parts and expressed this in a law of correlation.[2] Two weeks later, at 2 ; 0, 18, " Mama " is only a circular scribble with two legs pointing upwards, and after a further month, 2 ; 1, 6, no more than the complicated tangle of a circular scribble. But in this last drawing we meet the first attempt to represent clothes. Margaret took the red pencil for the circular scribbling, and then drew a few curved lines over it with the blue pencil, and said that that was the dress.

These obvious relapses were due to the Spring and Summer days, in which hardly any drawing was done, while in Winter she drew almost every day. Some sketches preserved from the months of June and July are proof of the absence of any desire to represent anything whatsoever ; along with a little circular scribble we have nothing but the most primitive kind of wavy scribble. The first months of the third year were thus a period of degeneration.

A curious trait which characterized this period deserves mention. At 2 ; 0, 18, she drew a very good pole for a flag drawn by me, and she then placed beside the flag a few wavy lines, and drew quickly a long and bold stroke sideways, remarking " there goes the flag ". In order to test whether she really meant this, I asked her, " where does the flag go ? " " There," she said, and pointed to the line. She thus represents movement itself in the form of a line.

When Margaret again began to draw in the Autumn, her human formula consisted of a small circle in the middle, around which a complicated circular scribble is placed ; once, at 2 ; 4, 22, two strokes as legs also appeared. A month afterwards it was more successful ;

[1] F. Krueger, " Zur Einführung ". " Über psychische Ganzheit ". *Neue psychologische Studien*, 1, pp. 23 *et seq.* (1926).
[2] F. Seifert, " Zur Psychologie der Abstraktion und Gestaltauffassung ", *Ztschr. f. Psychologie*, 78, p. 109.

she drew a badly closed oval in a single stroke, in which

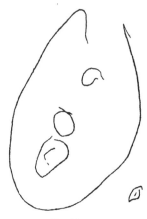

she set the eyes, for the first time, as circular rings; the arms and legs were missing. At 2; 5, 22, she drew herself in this fashion, both in a larger size with three large eyes, and in a smaller size with only one eye (Fig. 20).

At 2; 6, 29, we have the first attempt at the picture of a situation—Margaret on the sofa. The back of the sofa is given by a curved line, and a few straight lines beneath this, together with the cross lines at the side, produce a result some-what like the outline of a sofa;

FIG. 20.—BIG MARGARET AND LITTLE MARGARET. 2; 5, 22. 1/2.

but Margaret is only a circular scribble rounded in the

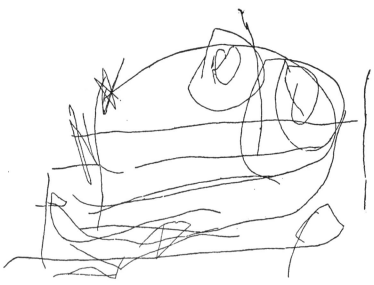

FIG. 21.—MARGARET ON THE SOFA. 2; 6, 29. ABOUT 1/2.

middle (Fig. 21).   At 2 ; 7, 6, she drew for the first time
a circle with two correctly placed eyes; this happened
two days after we had satisfied ourselves, for the first
time, that she had a clear conception of the number
two.

A few weeks later, at 2 ; 7, 20, she drew the portraits
of her father, mother, and nurse, and in doing so produced
a quite curious formula.   There is a circle with two eyes

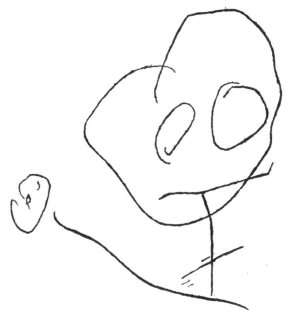

FIG. 22.—FATHER AND MOTHER.   2 ; 7, 20.   1/1.

and a mouth in fairly correct proportion ;   from the
head, and generally from the line representing the mouth,
a line goes downwards ;   across the lower part of which
a couple of lines, or a zig-zag scribble, are drawn.   Whether
these represent legs, arms, or clothes is not certain
(Fig. 22).   On the same day she repeated this formula
as a scribbling exercise at least thirty times, along with
other scribble ;   in her hurry the mouth often appears

over the eyes (Fig. 23). In spite of frequent repetition in the time following, this formula also disappeared as the previous two, fairly correct ones, had done. At 2 ; 7, 20, she drew a number of small lines on the paper and said : "All the people walking in the street."

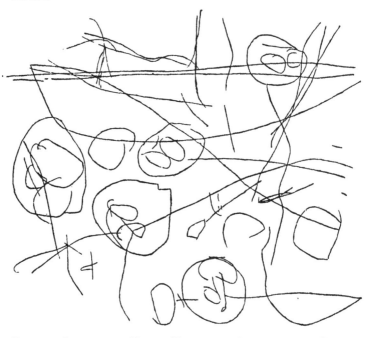

FIG. 23.—SCRIBBLE OF HUMAN HEADS WITH INDICATIONS OF BODY LINES. FROM MARGARET'S DRAWING. FRAGMENT. 2 ; 7, 20. ABOUT 2/3.

In place of the flag and the flower, Margaret chose in this Winter two new objects for drawing, the electric tramway and the railway. Both of them, but particularly the electric tram, had to be drawn for her again and again, and she was also very much attracted by a picture of a tram in her picture-book. She could not of course read, but she often looked at the pictures, and we had to tell her what was written. There now appeared the curious phenomenon observed in the previous Winter, viz., a series of industriously repeated and apparently intentional exercises with the object of being able to draw the tram.   She drew rectangles and divided them by a cross into four equal parts, or by shorter cross lines into smaller irregular parts ; she drew long lines with cross lines and thus again obtained straight or elongated rectangles.   Now and then she placed circles in a regular manner in each of the four rectangles.

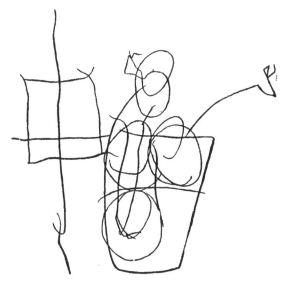

FIG. 24.—SCRIBBLE. PRACTICE FOR TRAM. 2 ; 8, 27. 1/2.

Some examples at the age of 2 ; 8, 27, are given in Fig. 24. For a few months her drawing retained this character almost exclusively, and may be best described as a kind of ideomotive rectangular scribbling, produced by mental pictures of forms and form elements, which had been impressed upon her by the tram and the railway being frequently drawn for her.   When I once asked her what it was, she answered definitely, "It's nothing."

In this period, she made from time to time, conscious

attempts to draw the trams ; some of them are reproduced here. At 2 ; 7, 20, the tram is produced for the
first time and repeated (Fig. 25) ; Figs. 26 and 27 were

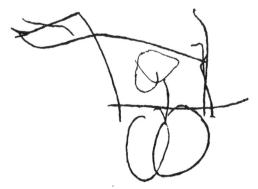

FIG. 25.—THE TRAM. 2 ; 7, 20. 1/1.

produced at 2 ; 8, 13, and 2 ; 8, 27, respectively. Fig.
28, at 2 ; 9, 13, is the most successful. The rectangle,
although she had made a better one before this, is fairly
regular, the wheels are worse than in the previous draw-

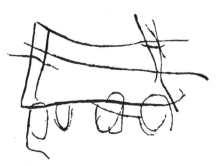

FIG. 26.—THE TRAM. 2 ; 8, 13. 1/1.

ings, and over the whole we see the sloping trolley-
pole which she called " the Klingeling " since she believed
that it was used to sound the bell. In the carriage
she has drawn herself.

She also asked several times for the flag and the flower. At 2 ; 11, she tried the flag herself, but only managed a few angles and crossed lines. At 2 ; 11, 2, her representation of a human being is a circular scribble with two lines as legs. The last drawings kept of the end of the third year are only scribbles, including even some wavy scribbling. In the last two months she had hardly done any drawing, perhaps on account of another kind of amusement, which she was offered since the Autumn.

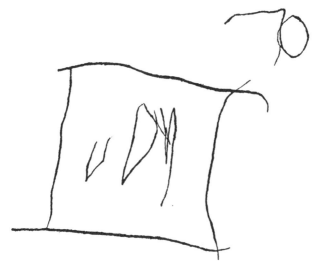

FIG. 27.—THE TRAM. 2 ; 8, 27. 1/1.

This was the cutting out of paper figures, which may further have been of some importance in regard to her development in the direction of comprehending forms. In this case, also, she continually asked for the same figures, a large and a small paper man which she calls " Big Man " and " Little Man ". In this connection an amusing example òccurred of the child's clinging to the traditional (at 2 ; 9) ; " Big Man " and " Little Man " had been cut, whereupon the idea occurs to her : " Take off hat!" I then cut off the " Big Man's " hat from

his head. She looked at the hatless head discontentedly
for a little while and then said : " Cut hat on again."
Since I had good reason for not being able to do this,
she passed me the scissors and said insistently : " Cut
hat on again." As far as I know she never tried to cut
figures herself, although she often cut paper up.

Margaret had done less drawing in the third year than
in the second year, and also made less progress. Nevertheless, she was still ahead of most of the six children
whose drawings have been closely observed. Her draw-

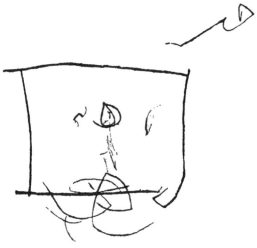

FIG. 28.—THE TRAM. 2 ; 9, 13. 1/1.

ings of the tram show a firmer and clearer line and better
form than the locomotives of Walther-Heinz Dix, who
drew best of these six children. The limitation to a
few motives is common to both. On the other hand,
Major's boy attempted several motives, usually, however,
when he was asked for them and mostly only from
copies ; one of these was the locomotive, which at three
years he still produced formlessly and badly. The same
is true of his attempts to draw an elephant, a dog, etc. ;
for even in his thirty-sixth month they have no similarity

to what had been drawn as examples for him, and it
was impossible to guess from them what they were
meant to represent. At 3 ; 0, he made a very bad
attempt to draw a rectangle, and produced only an
irregular oval with a line crossing it. It is surprising
that this reproduction of something drawn for him
failed so completely, for Walther-Heinz, like Margaret,
drew from memory quite neat and regular rectangles.
It is not impossible that the system of drawing instruction
and examples used by Major in the case of his son, may
rather have hindered than helped the boy's natural
aptitude for drawing. It has long ago been shown that
a child's drawing in the first period is almost exclusively
a matter of memory, and that it draws best when it is
allowed free play to reproduce its ideas.

Scupins' child, at the age of three, had also not made
very much progress. He used his formula, a circle with
two lines, to designate a lantern ; two rings are round
windows ; once he drew a rabbit, that somewhat recalls
the outline of a sitting rabbit ; at one end of this he
placed a small tangle of lines for the eyes. At 2 ; 11,
11, he drew a little boy. These were his productions in
the third year.

If we compare the formulæ of the seven children for
the human form, Margaret's peculiar formula at 2 ; 7,
20, is about as good as that of the others. Excepting
in one case where he drew his father with head, body
and legs, and even with a top-hat and a boot, Walther-
Heinz only drew faces without bodies, with two circles
as eyes and a nose.[1] Bubi drew at 2 ; 11, 11, a " Bubi "
—a circle, two legs, two arms, but only when asked
did he put in the features.[2] Major's boy drew on the
last day of the third year a circular scribble with two
lines as legs, two for arms, and a few small scribbles
for hair and ears.[3] Ekki, on the other hand, has already
drawn at this age a number of different human formulæ,

[1] Dix, *loc. cit.*, p. 75.   [2] Scupin, *loc. cit.*, pp. 199, 263.
[3] Major, *loc. cit.*, pp. 57, 59.

the latest having eyes, nose, mouth, hair, arms and legs, and even coats and buttons.[1] Günther and Simonne only succeeded in producing formalized drawing after completing the third year.

THE FOURTH YEAR

Margaret did less drawing in her fourth year than in her third. At first she continued to practise rectangles, some of which were larger than formerly. The usual Summer break commenced, however, earlier in this year, and continued longer into the Autumn than usual. Other observers have also noticed that children give up drawing completely, particularly in the Summer months, taking it up again with renewed energy afterwards. Stern, for example, speaks of a pause of nine months in the drawing of his son in the fourth year.[2] Dix mentions a seven-months' pause in Summer in the case of Walther-Heinz.[3]

When Margaret began to draw again in the Autumn, she had acquired a new taste—she drew letters, it being the large Roman letters which she tried to acquire at the age of three and a half years. As far as I can tell, she has never tried to draw other letters than those, the shape and sound of which were known to her. She had no actual teaching, but asked from time to time what the name of this or that letter was, or asked to have drawn for her a letter which she knew but could not draw. Sometimes she received a more systematic lesson in a playful fashion.

At 3 ; 8, 17, she drew O E L H, H and O being so large that they took up a whole sheet of paper, while most of the others were drawn of moderate size (Fig. 29). E, H, L and O were drawn horizontally instead of vertically, at an angle of about 30° to the horizontal and also in mirror writing. This imperfect representation has been called spatial displacement ; it is often met with in the

[1] Krötzsch, loc. cit., p. 76.   [2] W. Stern, loc. cit., pp. 5, 6, 13.
[3] Dix, loc. cit., p. 79.

earliest children's drawings and in the first attempts of children to write figures and letters.

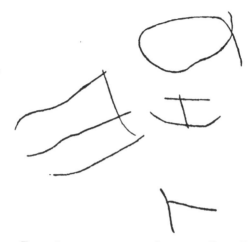

FIG. 29.—FIRST ATTEMPTS TO DRAW LETTERS. BLUE PENCIL. 3 ; 8, 17. 1/2.

Margaret's drawings also confirm the fact that spatial displacement is particularly characteristic of the first beginnings. At first her letters are horizontal, but in a week, at 3 ; 8, 25, the four or five letters which she can draw already appear in their correct positions (Fig. 30). Simultaneously with the first letters, at 3 ; 8, 17, a curious scribbling appeared. She divided a large sheet of paper by a cross in the middle, correctly calling it "cross", and then filled the paper with long lines of rounded zig-zags and said that they were "mountains" (Fig. 31). She probably did not intend to draw mountains ; the interpretation

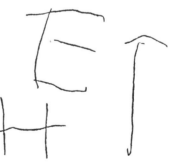

FIG. 30.—LETTERS. 3 ; 8, 25. 1/2.

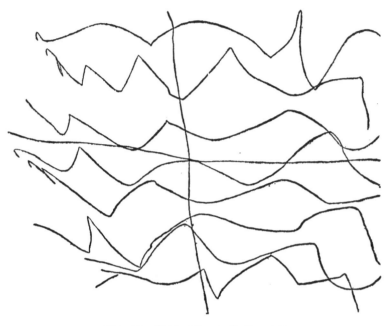

FIG. 31.—SCRIBBLE. 3 ; 8, 17. 1/2.

was no doubt an afterthought suggested by the similarity
of the lines to mountain tops. At 3 ; 8, 27, dense
masses of wavy scribbling were produced together with
letters (Fig. 32).

The last months of the fourth year were signalized by
another pause in her drawing. In this Winter also, she

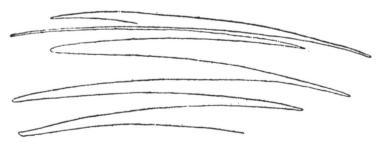

FIG. 32.—WAVY SCRIBBLE. FRAGMENT. 3 ; 8, 27. 1, 2.

displayed a love for cut-out paper figures, and, as at the earlier period, she demanded continual repetition of the same figure ; she now said " cut out little girls " : namely, a circle of little girls, and best of all, with a Christmas tree in the middle. She also asked for the " Bukkene Bruse ", the Troll and the bridge [1] and other subjects such as horses, bow-wows, bears, and man. This cutting-out of fairy-tale pictures was perhaps a preparation for the next phase of her drawing.

THE FIFTH YEAR

Margaret's drawings once again changed their character in the next year of her life ; they now became chiefly imaginative. Her drawings were, in fact, to an increasing degree the expression of mental pictures, particularly imaginative ones ; either she drew, in order to put on paper something she had pictured in imagination, or else she imagined a content for a drawing already executed. She frequently ascribed to a part of the drawing, while she was actually engaged in making it, a new meaning, on account of some chance similarity of form ; the new meaning then determined for her the next part to be drawn, and this might then also be given a fantastic meaning.

In this way the final drawing may represent something quite different from what she set out to draw. This does not disconcert her ; on the contrary, she finds great pleasure in this play of the imagination. The quick change of forms and pictured images suggests that her ideas are fugitive, and is in strong contrast to the rigid persistence with which she used to demand the endless repetition of one or two given drawings. The same fanciful change in motive was observed by Major in the case of his son [2] and by Dix [3] in the case of Walther-Heinz at about 4 ; 8, i.e., also in the fifth year. Stern also observed it in the case of his son Günther at about

---

[1] A Norwegian folk-tale.   [2] Major, *loc. cit.*, pp. 52, 53.
[3] Dix, *loc. cit.*, p. 85.

4 ; 0.[1] Scupins in Bubi's case in the fifth year,[2] and Luquet in the case of Simonne.[3]

As usual, a pause in drawing followed in the Summer half of the year. But when she by chance once got hold of paper and pencil in the holidays at 4 ; 3, 21, she made an attempt which was much bolder than any of her previous efforts, a very difficult problem indeed, namely, drawing a girl on a swing (Fig. 33). Swinging

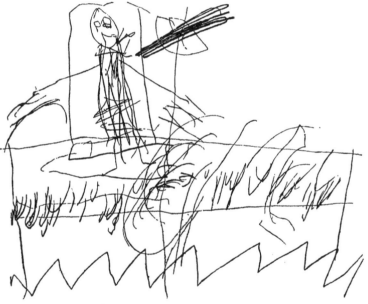

Fig. 33.—A little Girl swinging. 4 ; 3, 21. 1/2.

was one of her favourite amusements at this time, hence the mental picture of it was very much alive and ready to hand. She drew the swing beginning with one rope, following this with a sharp angle and making the seat in the same stroke, carrying on with the rope on the other side, and joining the two ropes at the top. The girl

---

[1] Stern, loc. cit., pp. 7 et seq.   [2] Scupin, loc. cit., p. 120.
[3] Luquet, loc. cit., pp. 44 et seq.

is drawn freely suspended in the air in the middle, but in such a way that the legs project a little under the seat ; the head is a circle with eyes, a nose drawn as a circle, and a mouth ; a long body is filled in with shading, and the short legs each have cross strokes as feet. The arms stretch out far over the rope, and have five long strokes for fingers which are not connected with one another or with the arm. The body is completed above and below with a horizontal line, there is also a sort of neck. We thus have a very complete human formula. Under the whole we see a rectangle enclosed by lines, which she calls the earth, into which she puts the grass. This is the first time that the line or rather surface of the ground was produced. Apart from her attempt in her second year to draw herself in a tram, this was her first picture of a situation. The swing and the whole affair are drawn from memory, formalized it is true, but copied from reality as she observed it.

On the same day scribbling occurred, with straight strokes all about in one direction, zig-zag lines, and well-defined, drawn-out spirals in long loops (Fig. 34). All the lines were placed regularly and symmetrically on the paper and produced the effect of ornament.

A month later, at 4 ; 4, 28, the human form again appears, badly carried out ; the body is " open ", nose and mouth are missing, the fingers are shown as in the previous drawing. She criticized her own drawing : " I cannot draw it any differently (referring to the leg) : only Father can draw things like that " (sticking out her own leg).

A bear and a monkey were drawn on the same day, making use of the human formula, as children often do, when attempting to draw animals. The bear and the monkey are standing upright, no doubt under the influence of a picture-book where the animals, bear, lion and monkey, were shown upright and dressed like humans (Fig. 35).

At 4 ; 6, she made her first distinctly imaginative

drawing, a boat as seen from above ; the cross lines
no doubt represent the seats.   She finally drew a tangled

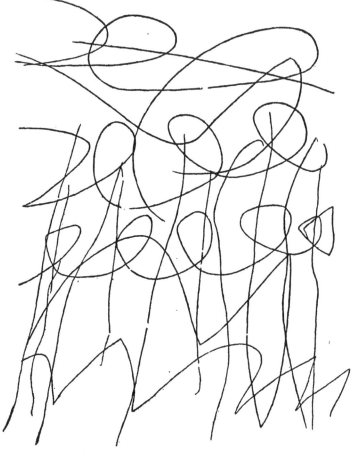

FIG. 34.—SCRIBBLE.   FRAGMENT.   4 ; 3, 21.   ABOUT 3/5.

circular scribble and said : " The *fjord* goes over it "
(Fig. 36).

Another drawing was prefaced by a triangle, said to
be a letter G, then two long strokes : " a boy's legs " ;
when she saw how long they were she called them front

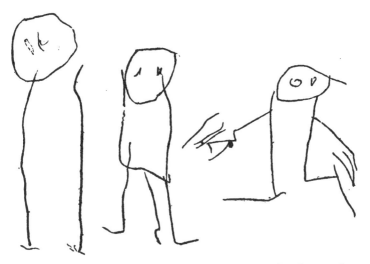

FIG. 35.—BEAR, MONKEY, AND HUMAN BEING. 4 ; 4, 28. ABOUT 3/5.

poles (flag poles ?) but then stood by the " legs " and drew a head with eyes on it, looked at it, changed the " legs " to " arms " and put a couple of further strokes as " legs " underneath it. She then made a circular scribble over

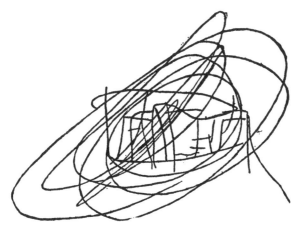

FIG. 36.—BOAT, " THE FJORD GOES OVER IT ". RED PENCIL. 4 ; 6. 2/3.

the whole and said : " The *fjord* came over him " (Fig. 37). After which she drew a ladder and zig-zag lines.

At 4 ; 6, 3, she drew "panes". She drew in one stroke a long line over the whole paper, and after she had drawn four long and fairly straight lines, she divided these with short cross-strokes into rectangles. She showed a sense of true proportion ; the distance between the strokes is approximately equal. She also tries to put the cross-strokes at equal distances, and when the distance apart is too great, she put an extra line in between (Fig. 38).

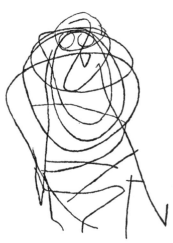

FIG. 37.—IMAGINATIVE DRAWING. BLUE PENCIL. 4 ; 6. 1/2.

On the same day she made her first attempt at a decorative drawing. She had a red and blue pencil, and drew with them in a straight line, first a piece of red, then a piece of blue, and then red again, and so on. When I asked her what her object was, she replied : " Because it must be pretty " (Fig. 39, see Plate facing p. 58). This was therefore a case of ornament in its simplest form of straight lines in various colours, repeated rhythmically, with the object of " making it pretty ". It is quite certain that no one had ever drawn ornament for her ; she may of course have observed it here and there, but certainly never in this form. Her ornament, extremely simple and primitive, appeared to spring from an original, primitive sense for the decorative.

Comparative research into the art of children and of primitive peoples has shown that illustrations are to be found very early in the art of individuals and in that of humanity.[1] This is also confirmed by Margaret's drawings. The next of her drawings which was kept, at 4 ; 6, 11, shows her attempting the problem of illustrating " The Wolf and the Seven Kids " (Fig. 40). She drew first the wolf, the largest figure ; she drew a rectangle, then the legs, first three and then another one, and afterwards the head. Then came the doubtful question : " Has he arms ? " I did not answer. She put on the left side a line pointing outwards and said : " That is the tail." Afterwards she drew the smallest figure to represent " White Fur ", one of the kids. But

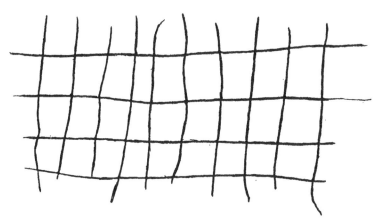

FIG. 38.—PANE SCRIBBLE. BLUE PENCIL. 4 ; 6, 3. ABOUT 2/3.

when she had finished it, she said : " That's a person, that's Red Riding Hood." It now becomes " Little Red Riding Hood ". Her " person " now had all the features on its face and no " open body ", but the fingers have disappeared and only appeared some months afterwards.

At 4 ; 6, 29, Margaret drew a " lady ", following the formula of her " Red Riding Hood ", but with an " open body ". A fresh step in her progress appears in an attempt to draw a dress, in the form of enormous buttons stretching in a long row from the head to the foot (Fig.

[1] Chamberlain, *The Child*, p. 203.

41). Psychologists who have studied drawing have observed that children pay particular attention to buttons, so that their drawing of clothes begins with these as the first and most important component. According to Lena Partridge, more than half their formalized humans, even when they have no clothes, are provided with buttons.[1] It is difficult to say why, unless we ascribe

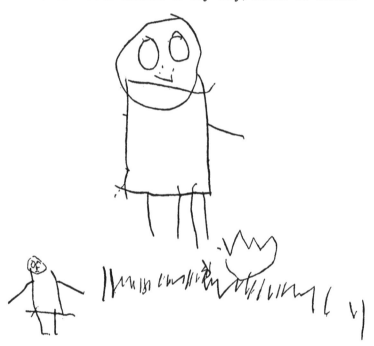

FIG. 40.—THE WOLF AND RED RIDING HOOD. 4 ; 6, 11. ABOUT 1/2.

it to the fact that buttons are comparatively easy to represent by a small circle, that is to say, by a shape easily mastered by the young artist.

At 4 ; 8, 22, Margaret's first house is produced in the following curious fashion. She drew a large rectangle, divided it into four other rectangles, and called it a

[1] Lena Partridge, *Children's Drawings of Men and Women*, pp. 171, 172.

" window ". " Shall I draw the house ? " she asked.
She did not then draw it, but instead made the window
into a house, drawing over it a triangle, " the roof ",
really the gable, and provided this with three small

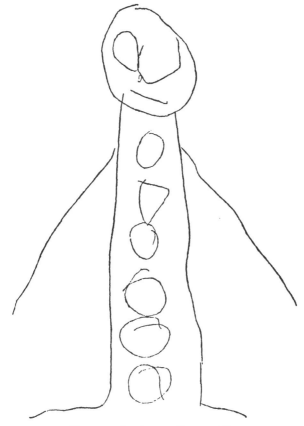

FIG. 41.—LADY. 4 ; 6, 29. 1/2.

windows. " Shall I draw the people living in it ? " she
then proposed, and there now appeared in one of the
upper panes of what had originally been the window
a human being : " Eyes, nose, mouth, buttons. That
is the lady of the house, two buttons on her blouse."

"How far does the blouse go?" I asked. "So far," she said, pointing to the lower edge of the pane and adding: "we don't see the rest, it's down there" (Fig. 42).

She thus knew already that the near covers the further away, and that this must be represented in a drawing.

On the same day she executed one of her elaborate imaginative drawings (Fig. 43). She first drew a circle in the middle and called it a "nought". But after

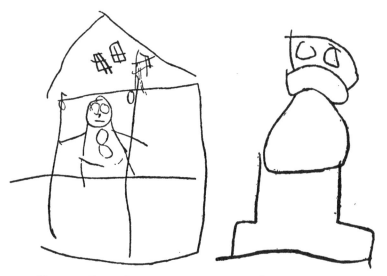

FIG. 42.—FIRST DRAWING OF A HOUSE. 4; 8, 22. 1/2.

FIG. 43.—IMAGINATIVE DRAWING. BLUE PENCIL. 4; 8, 22. 2/3.

looking at the shape thus produced, she said: "It's a coffee-pot." She then put a handle on the coffee-pot, looked at it, and said: "No, it's a lady with a flat head." She then forgot the head—the handle—was already there, and drew another head with eyes over it. She then took the legs in hand: "Just look what ugly legs she has." She joined the legs beneath with a cross-stroke; the form thus produced reminded her of the handle of a perambulator and she continued: "The lady is lying in a perambulator, they are pulling it here, she is lying in a fur." This in the same outline, all these different things, a nought, a coffee-pot, a fur, a lady, a perambulator, were imagined, and finally combined to form an impossible picture—a lady lying in a perambulator.

In this we have a picture of the child's manner of thinking and forming images in the first years of its life.

In the same way the child combines within the same word or concept the most various things, if they have but the slightest likeness to one another, or any single common point of contact which can serve to associate them in the child's mind. At 1 ; 5, for example, Margaret saw some specimens of butterflies on pins ; she called them flowers and tried to smell them as she usually did flowers ; another time she saw a picture of a tree and called it a flower. A flower, a butterfly, a

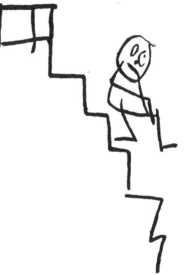

Fig. 44.—" A LITTLE GIRL CLIMBING UP TO HEAVEN." BLUE PENCIL. 4 ; 8, 22. ABOUT 2/3.

tree were combined under the concept " flower ".

On the same day, at 4 ; 8, 22, she drew a long staircase and said that it went up to heaven. Continuing : " There is a little girl climbing up to heaven." She looked at the legs, which were drawn crooked, and said : " Her legs are like that, because she is tired "—doubtless because she had climbed up many steps of this Jacob's Ladder (Fig. 44). Later on she again repeated the long staircase reaching to heaven. " Where shall we get to up

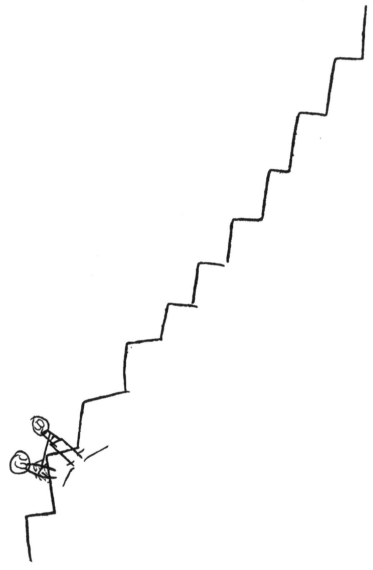

FIG. 45.—God carrying a Soul up to Heaven. Blue Pencil.
4 ; 8, 22. About 3/4.

there ? " I ask. " Up to God." She drew a person on
the staircase and said : " That's a dead man climbing
up to heaven." After a while she continued : " God is
carrying him up it," and drew a figure on the next step :
" That is God. He is taking him on his arm." Whereupon she made an arm down to the first figure (Fig. 45).

She drew two parallel lines and called them telephone
wires, and followed this by drawing a strip covered with
shading, saying : " That's the road, it's very long."
She then drew, in firm and clear strokes, dense masses
of circular scribbles, mostly ovals, wavy lines and curved
lines, with regular forms and clear, firm strokes.

At 4 ; 9, Margaret drew a lady with a blouse and
skirt. Having done this, the shape of the skirt reminded
her of a wash-tub, whereupon she put a handle on either
side and said : " That was a lady doing washing." After
that a number of rectangles appeared around the wash-
tub, which represented the washing, which we are thus
able to see through the side of the wash-tub. She did
not find anything unlogical in this ; but her sense of
logic was offended by the fact that one of the buttons
of the blouse was visible underneath the edge of the
wash-tub, so she explained this by saying : " That is
a button which has fallen down " (Fig. 46).

Although Margaret had given a proof a week before,
that she knew very well that the nearer covers the more
distant, she made here—but only once or twice again—
a mistake quite generally found in children's drawings,
namely, drawing things not visible to the beholder. It
is possible that she intended this drawing to represent
a view from above into the wash-tub—in which case,
the mistake would be only one of perspective.

At 4 ; 9, 7, Margaret drew a table and a chair as
seen from the side, in single lines ; the table is only
a rectangle, and the whole stands upon a ground line
(Fig. 47). On the same day she produced a man, who
is dressed, for the first time, in a jacket, indicated by
two curved lines. " Three buttons." The fingers were

named out aloud while she was drawing; "thumb",
and so on, etc. Her human formula is thus becoming

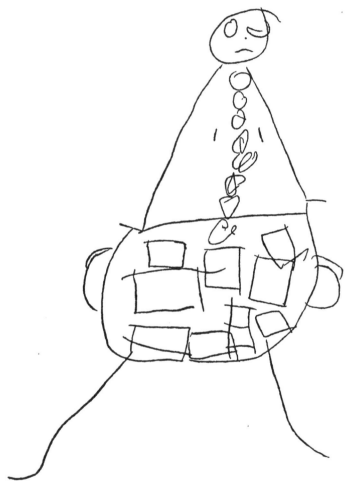

FIG. 46.—A LADY WASHING. RED AND BLUE PENCIL. 4; 9. 1/2.

differentiated; she drew, as we have said, a lady or girl
with a blouse and skirt, and a man with a jacket; the
latter, by the way, only occurs this single time (Fig. 48).

'When she had drawn the face of the man and noticed the turned-up corners of the mouth, she asked : " That's cheerful, isn't it ? "

Here we touch upon a debatable point in the psychology of children's draw- ing. Sully thinks that he finds in the formalized d r a w - ings of small chil- dren the expression of the most various

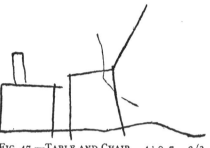

FIG. 47.—TABLE AND CHAIR.   4 ; 9, 7.   2/3.

moods : grinning rudeness, intoxicated joy, mad excite- ment, and so on.[1]   Others, such as Kerschensteiner and Bühler, think that Sully is completely wrong.   The drawings of a child are in reality, they think, stiff and expression- less : " The same formula is used to represent a funeral procession or a snowball fight."[2]   Bühler even says : " The important fact, that even the lines themselves, by means of their form alone, may be used for the direct expression of moods and mental excitement, is completely unknown to the average child at the first stage of drawing."[3]   Margaret's interpre- tation of the turned-up line of the mouth as cheerfulness shows, nevertheless, that this fact is already beginning to dawn upon her.   However, it is clear that she only reached this interpretation when the line had taken this form by pure chance.

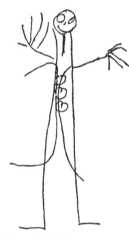

FIG. 48.—MAN.   4 ; 9, 7.
1/2.

[1] Sully, *Studies of Childhood*, p. 397.
[2] Kerschensteiner, *Die Entwicklung der zeichnerischen Begabung*, Munich, 1905, p. 17.
[3] Bühler, Eng., Tr. *The Mental Development of the Child*, London, 1933.

At 4 ; 11, 13, Margaret's human formula acquired teeth. For this purpose the mouth line is widened into a capacious oval, which is filled up with two rows of terrifying canine teeth produced by a pair of zig-zag lines. At the same time, ears appear for the first, and for the present only time, in the form of two large circular scribbles standing out on each side of the head. The buttons are drawn this time as spiral lines. " He has

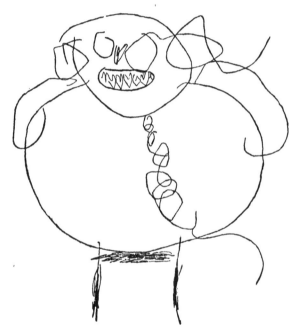

FIG. 49.—MAN. 4 ; 11, 13. 1/2.

no legs," she said ; " he is sitting on a chair." The drawing is done rapidly and rather carelessly (Fig. 49). On the same day she did some zig-zag scribbling with clear lines.

The last drawing preserved from the fifth year, at 4 ; 11, 20, is an attempt to imitate ordinary handwriting (Fig. 50).

She scribbled short lines of small, dense, zig-zag shapes and loops on paper ; afterwards she asked the question : " What is that ? " In her opinion this writing, if made to look as nearly as possible like the original, must also mean the same thing as the writing of grown-ups.

Margaret's drawing developed rapidly and richly in the fifth year, particularly as compared with her progress in the third and fourth year. She must have acquired a certain control over the movements of her hands and by no means a small degree of power to produce the line, since she was able to give a quick and bold expression to the most various constructions and mental pictures. Her drawings became more differentiated, primitive as

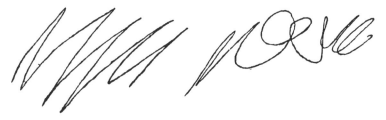

FIG. 50.—SCRIBBLE. IMITATION OF HANDWRITING. 4 ; II, 20. ABOUT 5/6.

they are ; they show the first beginnings of realistic drawing and fantastic drawing, of ornament and illustration ; her human formula develops and gains in detail. The most characteristic trait is, that the drawings now have a much higher degree of intellectual content, and reproduce the rapid change of her ideas in fantastic and sometimes even adventurous and impossible combinations.

Her drawings give us an account of her mental development : increased fertility of ideas and increasing capacity for bringing these in relation to one another, a more rapid play of ideas, a greater imaginative activity, and also, at the same time, a want of leading ideas and consecutiveness.

In the sixth year, Margaret's drawing lost its fantastic character, and became more realistic. Its leading characteristic may now be best stated as that of composition, in the most primitive sense of the word. She put letters together to form words, and drew mainly situation pictures. As opposed to her past year, her trains of ideas are no longer fantastic and casual, but are influenced by leading motives.

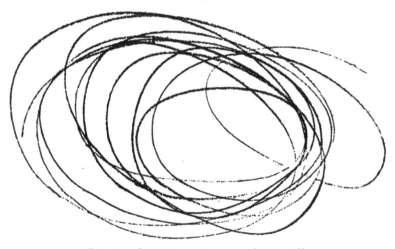

FIG. 51.—SCRIBBLE. 5 ; 2, 13. ABOUT 5/6.

As usual, little drawing was done in the first half of the year. A few pages have been preserved from June at 5 ; 2, 13. The scribble on one of these produces an almost æsthetic impression. A few beautiful and regular inter-linked ovals have been carried out with pure and accurate line (Fig. 51). The other shows an attempt to represent a book in an illustrated cover. The book is shown as a long narrow rectangle, and some distance away from it are two lines which she explained by saying, " That is what is underneath it." That is, she drew what was not to be seen, the leaves of the book and the lower side of the binding. She then continued : " Now I'll draw a picture ; there are pictures on it, you know." She drew on the cover a lady. This attempt at decorative art was thus principally a matter of imitation, and the coarsely and carelessly drawn lines of the feminine form cannot be by any means described as a success. Afterwards she explained a few chance characteristics : " She is fat." Regarding the arms, which are only shown by two projections, she said : " Those are arms, she's holding them like this "—pressing her hands to her side with her elbows sticking out. Underneath she drew instead of legs a sort of foot-piece, then looked at it and said : " Do you know what that is ? That's a wash-tub." Here we have a continuation of her imaginative interpretation of the year before (Fig. 52).

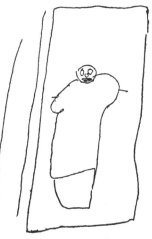

On the same day she drew a number of letters, as before Roman capitals : A, B, D, E, I, K, L, M, N, O, R, T, U ; an M standing on its head was rubbed out because it was " upside-down ", but

FIG. 52.—BOOK WITH ILLUSTRATION. 5 ; 2, 13. 1/4.

she did not notice that the N is likewise inverted (Fig. 53). She still has therefore a tendency to spatial displacement. She then asked me to draw for her some letters that she had forgotten : F, S, V.

At 5 ; 6, 24, she scribbled letters with pen and ink, and then made a wavy line and a line with rectangles open towards one side and the other ; both these produce the effect of an ornament (Fig. 54). She also drew zig-zag lines and a formalized human being, which is at last provided with hair shown as zig-zag lines ; the

body is " open ", there are buttons, but no arms. At
5 ; 7, 3, she drew on her own initiative FAR and MOR

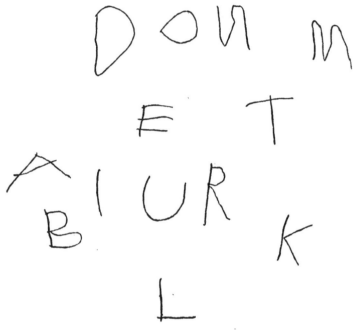

FIG. 53.—LETTERS. 5 ; 2, 13. ABOUT 1/2.

(Father and Mother, Fig. 55), and then a number of
other letters, and scribbles and straight strokes and
zig-zag lines.

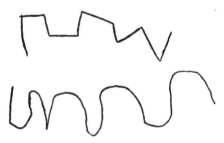

FIG. 54.—ORNAMENTAL SCRIBBLE. PEN DRAWING. 5 ; 6, 24. 1/2.

At 5 ; 8, 20, Margaret tried to draw a tree. First came the trunk, and then she stopped and thought, and then said : " I can't draw the bushes there, there

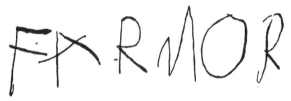

FIG. 55.—" FAR, MOR " '(FATHER, MOTHER). PEN. 5 ; 7, 3. 1/1.

should be some bushes there but I can't draw them." As I made no move to help her, she made after awhile a few curved uninterrupted lines which are supposed to represent the top of a tree (Brush formula, Fig. 56).

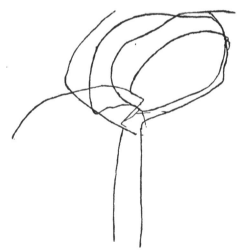

FIG. 56.—TREE. 5 ; 8, 20. ABOUT 3/4.

She then drew a flower with red and blue pencil. The flower itself looks like a tulip painted one half red and the other half blue, the beautifully curved stem carries on the one side a red, and on the other side a blue, leaf

in simple line ; underneath is the outline of a flower-pot.
When she was finished she said : " Isn't that pretty ? "
Here we must take account of decorative drawing ;
the colour is certainly decorative and not natural (Fig. 57,
see Plate). On the same day, at 5 ; 8, 20, she made
wavy and circular scribble.

At 5 ; 9, 6, a house in the form of a large rectangle
was produced, without a roof, and with three rows of
windows, which are decorated with curtains in sloping
wavy scribbling. The door is missing, but in one corner

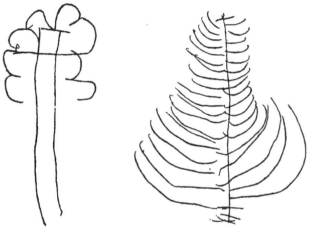

FIG. 59.—TREE. 5 ; 9, 6.   FIG. 60.—CHRISTMAS TREE. 5 ; 9, 7.
      ABOUT 3/4.   1/2.

is a staircase and underneath it " grass ". The drawing
shows only that characteristic of a town house, a wall
with many windows.

On the same day Margaret again drew a flower, which
looks rather like a small oak leaf with lobate edges, and
stem which continues as the central rib of the leaf. The
flower is red above and blue below and is placed in a
globular vase, one half red and the other blue (Fig. 58,
see Plate). She followed this with a tree, the crown of
which is represented in similar lobate outlines (lobate
formula). These she supposes to represent the leaves

(Fig. 59). On the next day she drew a Christmas tree. The branches are formed by single lines going out to either side, long below and shorter above, thus producing the usual aspect of a fir-tree (Fig. 60).

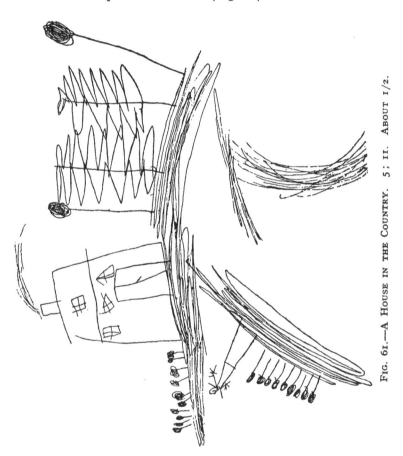

FIG. 61.—A HOUSE IN THE COUNTRY. 5 ; 11. ABOUT 1/2.

At 5 ; 11, she drew a " house in the country ". It has a roof with a chimney, only three windows; and a door. On the one side of the house there are trees ; some are carried out in broad dense zig-zag lines on both sides of the trunk, others have a tall trunk with a crown of very

dense circular scribble (coil formula).   On the other side
are flowers in a " button formula ".   The ground consists of shaded wavy scribble ; the path planted with
flowers leads up to the house.   On the path a man is
walking, whose feet are turned outwards.   This is the
first step towards representing human figures in profile,
and is like that of most other children.[1]   It is done from
the need of the moment, for the man must go to the
house, and hence she draws for the first time legs walking.
On the other side we see a waterfall in shaded lines,

slightly curved and pointing
downwards, a recollection of
the holiday resort (Fig. 61).

After she had been practising
latterly house, tree, flower, each
by itself, she now combined
them to a " landscape ", and
this fondness for composition
in the most elementary sense
of the word dominates her
future drawing.   On the same
day she drew a table with
chairs, and the " sun " (Fig. 62).

A " lady " was also pro-
duced.   After she had made
the two sloping lines outlining
the body, she drew by mistake,
on each side, a further sloping

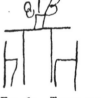

FIG. 62.—TABLE AND CHAIR,
AND THE " SUN ".   5 ; 11.
1/1.

line.   She first explained this as the lady stretching
out her coat, but later she discovers that it is a cape,
and thenceforward her ladies often appear with this
article of clothing.   The characteristic lines of the
cape were gradually drawn out into caricature, as in
one of the drawings of the following day (5 ; 11, 3 ;
Fig. 63).

On the same day, there appeared a curious house in
the form of a high and narrow triangle ; at the lower

[1] Krötzsch, *loc. cit.*, p. 80.

part a door and two windows, above a couple of cross lines, and between these again vertical lines, perhaps also representing a window. At the top a smoking chimney (Fig. 64). To a certain extent, this might represent the idea of a house seen from the gable end ; but it is really a kind of stylized, decorative house, which later on, since she finds it pretty and easy to draw, is used as " trimming " in her landscapes. This sup-

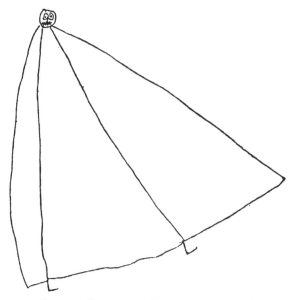

FIG. 63.—LADY WITH CAPE. 5 ; 11, 3. 1/1.

position appears to be confirmed by her own statement. At 6 ; 8, 8, when she had just drawn a house of this kind, I asked her : " Where have you seen a house like that ? " " I have never seen one like it." " Why do you draw it ? " " It's funny. I can't make any other kind." The last remark really means that another takes more trouble. Perhaps also the three-cornered cape shape which she was so fond of drawing at this time, may have had something to do with giving the house this form.

Nevertheless, we may take this as an example of spontaneous stylization which is very rare at this age ; indeed, Bühler maintains that it never occurs in the early drawings of children.[1]

She continued reading and drawing letters on her own initiative, and made from the letters she had practised words, and even whole sentences. Her progress is shown by "a letter to Father", which she undertook to draw at the age of 5 ; 11, 6. The contents are as follows : " father, dear, why are you so fond of Annemari, and Randi, and Laïla, and Elsie, and Tuppen and Lillemor and Vesleveste and Lillebagga and Dukkelise." Annemari and the others were her dolls. The bad spelling shows that this was entirely her own work. Underneath she drew all the dolls, all wearing capes (Fig. 65). The letter was put on the writing-table, so that her father might find it, and she asked her mother : " Don't you think that Father will be pleased ? " This is a proof of the fact that the art of a child, like all other art, is a matter of feeling ; she ascribes to her father the same feelings for her dolls which she has herself, and thinks that he must be just as pleased with her little work of art as she is herself.

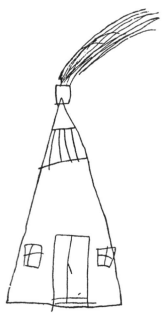

FIG. 64.—HOUSE. 5 ; 11, 3. 1/2.

At 5 ; 11, 7, Margaret drew a town house ; it differs from the country house in having a larger number of windows and chimneys. In the first storey there is a

[1] Bühler, *loc. cit.*, p. 167.

shop window with " oranges ", and a " chest " and a " lamp " above it. In the air there are birds flying, her first, and for a long time her only, attempt to

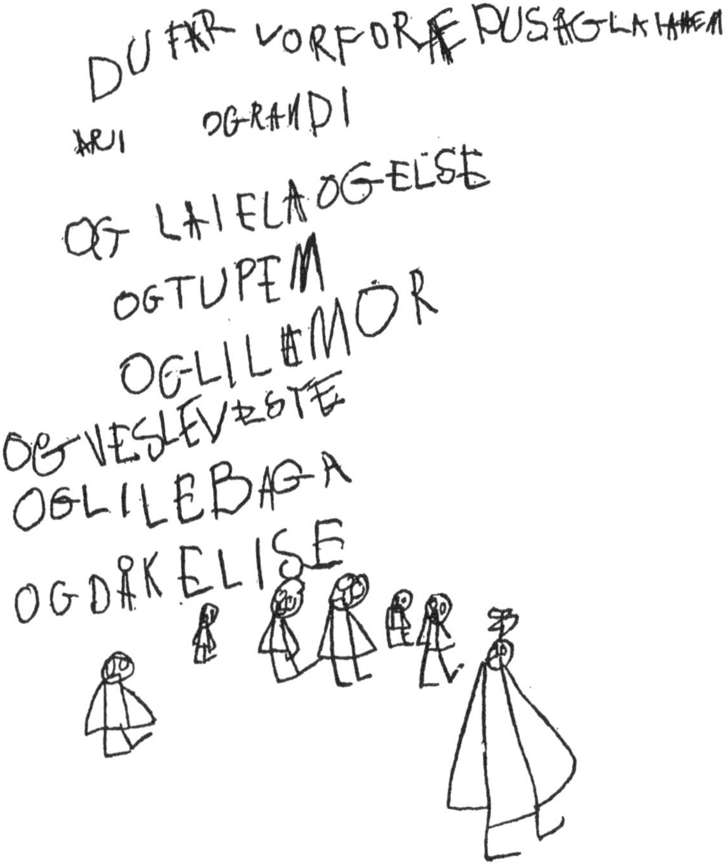

FIG. 65.—THE LETTER TO FATHER. 5 ; 11, 6. ABOUT 2/3.

draw birds ; the result, no doubt, of some external influence (Fig. 66).

At the age of 5 ; 11, 8, it appeared once more that she was very well aware of the want of agreement between her formalized drawings and reality. Pointing to the trees in the garden, she asked me to draw " a tree like that one over there ".

At 5 ; 11, 8, she drew " a woman on ski " : the ski are simple lines bent upwards ; she drew a few lines sticking out of the head in a haphazard manner, and then many more : that was the hair. " It is windy ",

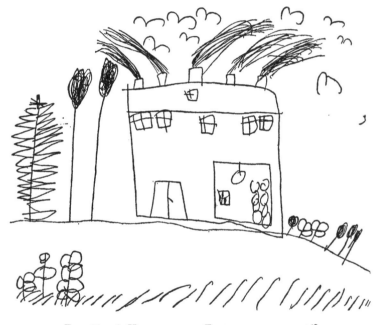

FIG. 66.—A HOUSE IN THE TOWN. 5 ; 11, 7. 5/8.

and the woman becomes a little girl with loose hair. At 5 ; 11, she had once before drawn a lady on ski.

On the same day she imitated with pen and ink ordinary writing, making long lines with strokes like writing, alternately resembling u's and e's. There are no long letters among them. I asked her what that meant and got as an answer : " Nothing " (Fig. 67). At the age of 5 ; 11, 13, she made long straight lines with the pen and drew letters on them, namely, an *e* in cursive and

a capital Roman R several times repeated regularly
spaced. These were followed by wavy lines and loops.

On the same day a situation picture was produced :
" All the dolls are tobogganing ". Some of the dolls

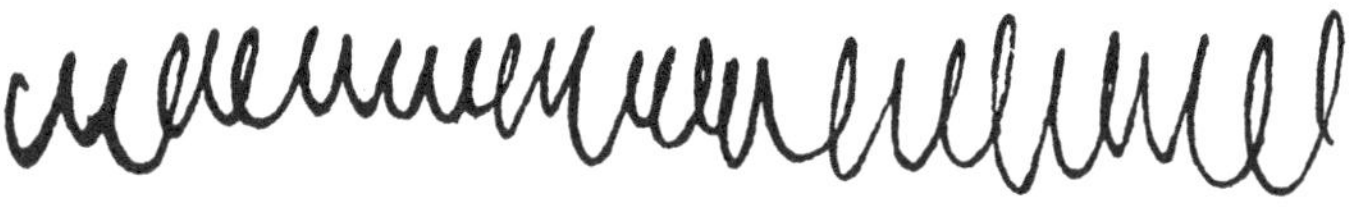

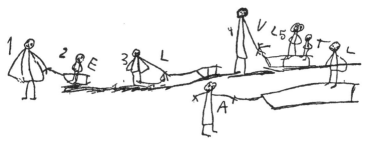

FIG. 67.—HANDWRITING SCRIBBLE. 5 ; 11, 8. PEN. 1/1.

are large, others small, some are pulling their sledges
behind them, and others are standing on their sledges ;
it was some months before she was able to draw a person
sitting. Alongside the dolls are the initial letters of

FIG. 68.—" ALL THE DOLLS ARE TOBOGGANING." RED PENCIL.
5 ; 11, 13. ABOUT 1/3.

their names, and they are also in part numbered, but not
beyond five because she had not yet practised the other
figures (Fig. 68). After this she drew her own name and
address. This was the last drawing of her sixth year.

THE SEVENTH YEAR

The four summer months of her seventh year, which
immediately preceded her first visit to school, did not
bring the usual pause in her drawing. She drew a great
deal, and exclusively compositions. Her drawings became more and more synthetic and logical, being the
expression of combinations of mental pictures and

P.C.D.   F

connected ideas. The representation was correct and true to nature to a degree somewhat greater than usual in the case of children of this age, although they retained a typically childlike character by reason of their formalized nature. The further development of her logical sense is shown above all by a new trait appearing in her seventh year, namely, the desire to produce correct perspective. She also begins to draw in outline.

The first picture of her seventh year, at 6 ; 0, 3, is a street picture, which has many points of interest (Fig. 69). Two ladies, each with a perambulator, meet in the street ; one perambulator is a push-cart, the other (in order to avoid monotony ?) a bassinette. The representation of both perambulators shows a curious attempt at perspective drawing, although in opposite directions. In the case of the push-cart, the cart itself, the handle, and the hood are in attempted perspective, although not of course correctly carried out ; the perspective of the hood was more successful in other drawings of perambulators, which now became a very favourite motive for her. Alongside this perambulator a small child is walking, holding on to the handle. When Margaret had just drawn this she asked me : " Do you see that the children—big children, walking alongside—are holding on here—on the handle—with the right hand ? " She appeared to be proud of her powers of observation, and often made use of this piece of realism. Behind the other perambulator two figures are walking. She explained these as follows : " Those are two children, of which we only see the head and the legs, because they are walking behind the bassinette." We have thus another characteristic of perspective drawing, namely, the crossing of lines. Three or four people walking, grown-ups and children, fill up the left half of the footpath. Between the two perambulators on the right there is a dog, and another right at the left, for the sake of symmetry or to fill up the empty space. This was her first attempt to draw animals since the fairy

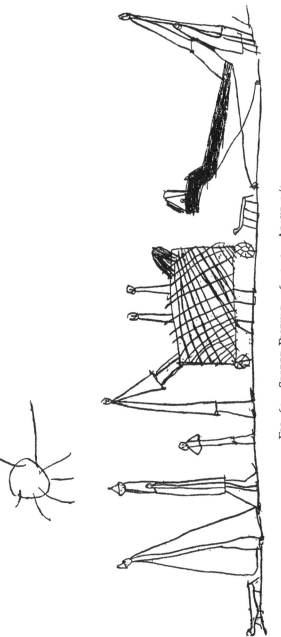

FIG. 69.—STREET PICTURE. 6 ; 0, 3. ABOUT 1/2.

story illustration, " The Wolf and Red Riding Hood ",
done in her fifth year.   Hence the more obvious mistakes
usually found in children's drawings had been avoided ;
seen from the side they are, apart from the equal spacing
of the four legs, drawn quite fairly well.   A further step
in progress in the matter of profile drawing is seen in
the arms drawn in profile, which were also the result of
the necessity for showing the pushing of the perambulator ; for the same reason the hands are shown in
circular scribble.   The wheels of the perambulators are
shown in absolute profile, for we only see the two visible
from the one side, although, judging by the perspective
of the hood and the handle, something of those on the
other side ought also to be seen.   Over the whole, the
sun is shining, a circle surrounded by rays.

While Margaret was in advance of her age in the
matter of perspective drawing, she makes in this drawing
the usual mistake of early children's drawings, namely,
the want of correct proportion.   Her human figures are
now much too long and have much too small heads.   As
some of these long, thin persons also have a pointed
cap on their heads, they look very much like street-
lamps, and such " lamp-post figures " now frequently
appear in her drawings.   Similar excessively long and
thin human figures have been found in the east of Spain
in rock paintings of the Stone Age.[1]

At 6 ; 1, 20, she drew a person sitting down for the
first time.   Margaret's conquest of this difficult piece
of representation was the result of chance.   She found
a piece of paper with a circle drawn on it, into which
she proceeded to place a nose, eyes and mouth.   She
then drew in haphazard fashion a bent line downwards
from the circle, whereupon the likeness to a person seated
struck her, and she added body and legs in the sitting
position (Fig. 70).   She immediately made use of her
new acquirement.   She first drew " Mother with Margaret

---

[1] H. Obermaier, " Paleolithikum und steinzeitliche Felskunst in
Spanien ", *Prähistorische Zeitschrift*, 13/14, p. 185.

on her lap " (Fig. 70) ; besides feet and arms we have
here for the first time the body drawn in profile.   The
mother's arms start both from one shoulder and are both
visible, but the way in which the mother holds Margaret
is correctly given, for one arm is hidden by Margaret's
body.   The hands are folded together with a circular
scribble.   She then draws Father and Mother and
Margaret on a sledge.   Here we have a new motive,

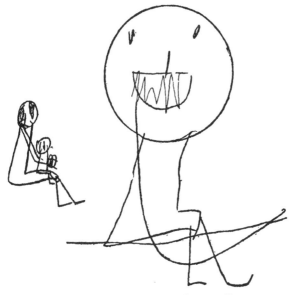

FIG. 70.—RIGHT : FIRST DRAWING OF A SITTING FIGURE.
LEFT : " MOTHER WITH MARGARET ON HER LAP." 6 ; 1, 20.

the hand-bag : " Father is looking after Mother's bag ".
She repeated this drawing with the sledge later on and
made other uses of her new power of representing sitting
positions.   She drew people sitting on a chair, and so
on.
    She often, about this time, imitated handwriting, and
now added also long loops, particularly below the line.
At 6 ; 1, 21, she asked me after she had scribbled a few

lines (Fig. 71) : " Is there anything right in it ? " When I then pointed to one or two signs which were like y and g, she asked me to write these letters for her, and then copied them. She practised industriously capital

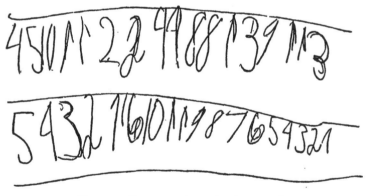

FIG. 71.—HANDWRITING SCRIBBLE. 6 ; 1, 21. 1/1.

Roman letters and numbers. At 6 ; 2, 8, it appeared that she had got as far as being able to write and read all figures from 1 to 11. She always wrote 11 in mirror writing, but 1 usually correctly (Fig. 72).

FIG. 72.—FIGURES. 6 ; 2, 8. ABOUT 2/3.

At 6 ; 2, 3, she made a drawing which again shows clear evidence of the effort to draw in perspective. We see Father, Mother and Margaret, tobogganing down a hill on sledges ; the path winds to-and-fro, so that one might imagine it to be intended for the well-known hill " The Corkscrew ". The path is drawn in perspective ;

below, where seen close to, it is broad, and gets narrower above, where it is further away. At the top of the picture is one of her three-cornered houses drawn very small, because it is far away (Fig. 73). On the previous day she made a remark which showed that she was conscious of drawing in perspective. She drew " a lady carrying a hand-bag " and said : " The head is here a little larger, because it is nearer "—than on a drawing she had just made.

At 6 ; 2, 20, we have a drawing, " the train ". The rails are drawn, but the train is not standing on them, but on one of the external lines. The locomotive has a door and windows like a house, and in the carriage windows many faces are seen. The lines run together towards the background in perspective ; right at the back is one of the above-mentioned triangular decorative houses, drawn quite small and with little detail (Fig. 74).

At 6 ; 2, 22, Margaret drew a garden scene. In the middle a table, and on it a flower, at each side a chair, each with a little girl sitting on it ; on both sides a flagstaff with a flag, one being the Norwegian flag, the other an imaginary flag. She began the picture by drawing the Norwegian flag. First she made the outline, then the blue cross with single strokes ; then she stopped and thought, for she did not know what the flag looked like : " What is it like ? " she asked, and was anxious that I should tell her. As I did not comply with the request, she thought for awhile, and then drew a red cross alongside the blue one. The flag and the whole garden scene were repeated two or three times in the next week in this form (Fig. 75, see Plate facing page 58).

This was a most instructive observation. The memory picture of a child may therefore be nebulous and incomplete to so great a degree. Who could ever have thought that she did not know what the Norwegian flag looked like ? She had a particular preference for it

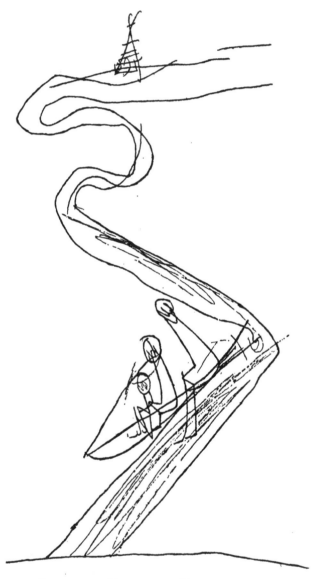

FIG. 73.—FATHER AND MOTHER AND MARGARET ON THE SLEDGE.
6; 2, 3. 1/1.

from her earliest childhood. Even at the age of two
to three years it had been drawn for her countless times
in its correct colours. On the 17th of May, she had
seen the procession of children with hundreds of flags ;
she herself possessed a small children's flag. One might
suppose that she 'had a particularly bad memory for

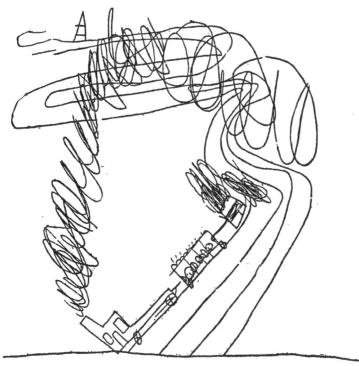

FIG. 74.—THE TRAIN. RED PENCIL. 6; 2, 20. ABOUT 5/9.

colours, but that is not true, for she knew the names of
all ordinary colours at the age of four. If her picture of
a shape which was so well known to her and had been
impressed upon her so many times, was so imperfect,
what can have been her pictures of things which she
had only seen a few times? In investigating children
attending school for the first time at the age of seven,

I also found their concepts in general unclear and poor in content.[1]

A new flag drawing, at the age of 6 ; 3, shows that it was the memory picture and not the ability to draw which was responsible for the failure. Margaret came running up with two small Norwegian flags, and set to work to draw them. We may suppose that she had seen the flags, had realized the incorrectness of her representation of them, and now wanted to draw a real flag. She had looked at them so closely that she had now become aware that there was white on them, and asked for " a white pencil ". She was given one together with a sheet of drawing-paper, and a red and blue pencil as well. She put one of the flags next to her and looked at it while she drew ; this is the first and only time that I have seen her draw from a model.

She first drew the blue cross with two double strokes, then the red areas with shading lines, and then tried to draw the white strips. When she saw that no colour was produced, she said angrily, " You can't see that," and gave it up. She left the blue cross only an outline, and did not fill it in with colour until I showed her how. (On a later occasion also, she left the cross in the drawing of the flag empty, although she coloured the surfaces around it.) Immediately afterwards she drew the outlines of the whole flag with red pencil, and last of all the flag-staff. Her procedure in this drawing was therefore synthetic, whereas children's drawings are normally characterized by the analytical method. Children generally draw the outline first and then the details.

Margaret then drew another flag and said : " I will draw two little girls sitting at their little table." She noticed that one of the girls was somewhat larger than the other, and said : " she's bigger, that is Gerd " (a small friend of hers) ; the other girl was Margaret. She then drew a huge sun. The large size was perhaps really

---

[1] Cf. Helga Eng, *Begynnernes forestillingskrets*, Oslo, 1923, pp. 40 *et seq.*

due to the cause given by her mother when she saw the drawing : " Yes, to-day the sun was very large." It was an unusually hot summer day, and Margaret had been out in the morning with her parents and had doubtless felt the power of the sun ; it is well known that children emphasize anything which has made a particular impression on them by representing it as very large. Next came a perambulator, pushed by Mother, with Margaret walking alongside and Father behind ; we do not see him. The three other figures have no names ; these, as also the perambulator, were quite certainly only drawn to fill up the picture, thus showing a certain degree of talent for composition (Fig. 76). She herself looked upon the picture as a work of art for she proposed : " Can't we hang it up with drawing-pins in the living-room ? " When I said that it wouldn't be suitable, she herself suggested a more suitable spot : " But in the nursery, I could have it there." In fact, she had altogether a high respect for her own drawings, and expected others to appreciate them ; the same is reported by Dix of Walther-Heinz.[1] At about the age of 6 ; 2, 25, she met with criticism for the first time. A ten-year-old little girl began to criticize her drawings and point out their mistakes, saying that they were ugly, and so on. Margaret turned dark red and her face assumed a curious expression. Surprise, humiliation, anger, and a certain amount of incredulity were indicated : it was unheard of —it could not be right—she kept silence, however. When the same child later on tore one of her drawings in two, she burst out crying and could only be pacified when I pointed out to her that she could draw another one, which she then did.

A drawing at the age of 6 ; 2, 21, shows the highest point reached in her representation of persons before she went to school. The figure lowest in the drawing is " Mother ". We see great progress in the representation of the dress ; the blouse is realistically drawn with the

[1] Dix, *loc. cit.*, p. 78.

cut of her mother's blouse correctly shown ; the sleeves
of the blouse are carried out in outline, but the arms and
legs are still single lines. The folds of the skirt are shown
by lines. The lady on the staircase is a " strange lady ".
" I beg your pardon," she said. " Why ? " " Yes,
because she is touching the hand of a strange lady "
(Fig. 77). Here again we have an explanation made to
fit, the hands having by chance been drawn close to-

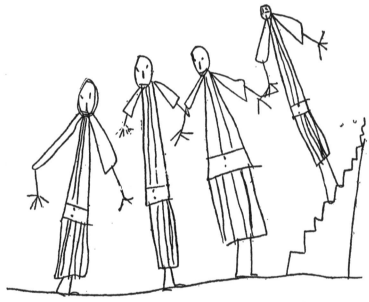

FIG. 77.—LADIES. RED PENCIL. 6 ; 2, 21. 2/3.

gether. We again see that the interpretation of posture
and gesture is not so foreign to children's drawings as
Bühler assumes.[1]

The figures show here good proportions as compared
with the long thin persons which she had drawn latterly.
At 6 ; 1, 13, she had made it clear that a conscious sense
of correct proportion was by no means wanting in her.
I put together a man with matches and set the arms

[1] Bühler, loc. cit., pp. 184, 185.

much too far down on to the body. She criticized : " The arms are not as low as that, the arms are up here " —whereupon she put them at the top of the man she had set out. " Are my arms like this ? " She pressed her arms to her side, stuck them out forward from the elbows, looked at me and laughed. " Don't you see that your arms are fixed on here ? "—grasping my arm at the shoulder. Part of the exaggeration and disproportion in her drawing, the " lamp-post " figures, " cape-figures " and others, may quite well indicate a certain preference for characterized exaggeration. Children's drawings are not quite innocent of conscious caricature, although their likeness to caricatures is frequently involuntary and the result of imperfect conception and technique. At 6 ; 3, 1, Margaret drew a man, and then suddenly put an enormously high hat on his head saying : " He has a Konfrutti hat." I do not know where she obtained the idea, and the expression ; if it was not her own invention she may have seen something comic of this kind somewhere. Then she drew a man and lengthened his arms, following a notion of the moment, down to the earth, and said : " That's an old man, he is walking with sticks." He also was given a pipe, quite by way of exception. The pipe usually plays, as Ricci remarks, an important rôle in children's drawings, particularly in the case of boys : " The pipe is the boy's highest ideal." Hence we find the pipe in all drawings, even the most primitive. " Look at this man : he consists of nothing but body and legs ; head and arms are missing. What does it matter since he is fortunate enough to possess a pipe ? " [1] In the case of the third figure the legs are rather a failure, which is explained by " his legs hurt him " (Fig. 78).

At 6 ; 3, 1, Margaret produced her last large com- position before going to school, one which best shows how far she had progressed in free and independent development of her single-line technique. In this case,

---

[1] Ricci, *loc. cit.*, p. 35.

by the way, we seek in vain for any attempt, such as is shown in earlier drawings, to draw in perspective. She said she would draw St. Hanshaugen, and began with what had the greatest attraction for her, namely, the swing. The swing was produced with its framework, a girl in the characteristic position of swinging, two little girls, one on either side, "waiting for their turn". Everything is correctly observed, and, as far as her primitive technique allowed, realistically represented;

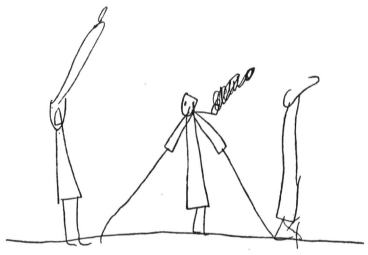

FIG. 78.—THE MAN WITH THE "KONFRUTTI HAT". A MAN WITH STICKS. "A MAN WHOSE LEGS HURT HIM". RED PENCIL. 6; 3, 1. ABOUT 1/2.

we are no longer dealing here with a mere formula, but with a little piece of reality. The blurring of the facial features is caused by the blue pencil and its thick lines. The swinging girl has arms to hold on with ; the two little girls, who have only to wait, do not need any arms.

Margaret now proceeded to change the scene, saying : " It's in the garden." She drew a clothes-line, suspended between two posts. On the line is hanging " washing ", " clothes ". and " knickers ". The clothes are drawn very neatly and correctly. There is trimming round the arms. This motive had already been especially practised earlier on. She was reminded of it this time by the form of the swing framework.

She then says, " Now I'll draw the house," and like lightning one of her triangular decorative houses appears on the free space at the left (Fig. 79).

The whole drawing was put on the paper quickly and energetically, and shows an astonishing mastery of line as a means of expression for a six-year-old child. A ruler set alongside the lines shows them to be creditably straight, although they were drawn freely in one stroke, and, for example, in the case of the house are about 12 centimetres long ; the triangular house is an almost regular equilateral triangle. The weakest point, in this as in her other drawing, is the careless way in which lines separately drawn are made to meet.

Considered as a picture, this drawing bears witness to a decided sense, whether instinctive or conscious, of harmonious composition ; even the smoke going from the house across the picture contributes to the unity of the whole.

When she finished, I reminded her that she wanted to draw St. Hanshaugen. " Then I must have a larger piece of paper," was the reply, " I have no room on this for all of it." After a little while, she continued : " I can't draw St. Hanshaugen, that's too difficult." Again a proof of self-criticism. It is also related concerning Walther-Heinz, Günther, and Simonne, that they exercised self-criticism, and even tore up drawings with which they were not satisfied.[1] On the same day she scribbled imitation handwriting and again asked : " Does that look like anything ? " The lines are now divided into single " words " ; some of the loops were made extremely long (Fig. 80).

At 6 ; 4, 2, she drew a dog-kennel, such as she had seen in the holidays in the country, and to this she

---

[1] Stern, *loc. cit.*, p. 16 ; Dix, *loc. cit.*, p. 69 ; Luquet, *loc. cit.*, p. 15.

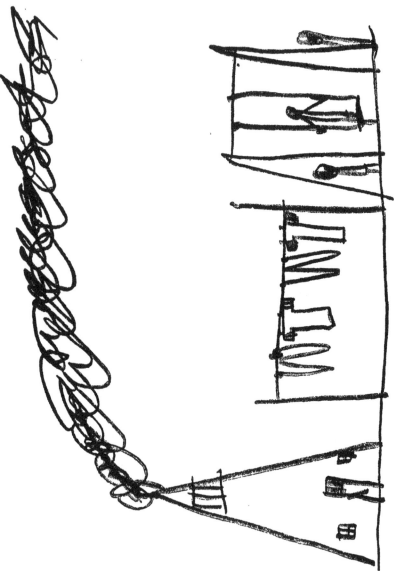
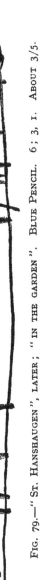

FIG. 79.—" St. Hanshaugen ", later; " in the garden ". Blue Pencil. 6 ; 3, 1. About 3/5.

added some details of an ordinary house. She then wished to draw the dog, and in order to make it as easy as possible she said, " We can only see its tail," and drew a line upwards in the entrance. But she then realized that the dog itself would be in an impossible position, and drew the tail at the bottom near the entrance. I then proposed that she should draw the whole dog, whereupon she produced it by sketching a human face with eyes, nose and mouth. This feature, which otherwise is fairly common in children's drawings, was only observed by me in her drawings on this single occasion. I pointed out to her that her dog had only two legs, whereupon she replied : " We don't see the other two." The two dogs' heads in the windows are

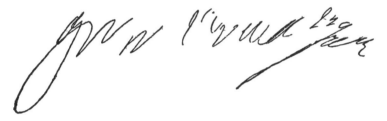

FIG. 80.—HANDWRITING SCRIBBLE.   PEN.   6 ; 3, 1.   ABOUT 1/2.

somewhat more realistic (Fig. 81). This is her last drawing before she went to school at 6 ; 4, 6.

At 6 ; 4, 8, she produced as part of a larger picture—triangular house, flag, clothes-line with washing—a pigeon-cote such as she had seen in the country (Fig. 82).

At 6 ; 4, 28, she produced a larger composition consisting of a house, according to the formula of 5 ; 11, 7, one of the traditional perambulators, together with (a new feature) a cart with horse and driver ; on the cart is written in her imperfect spelling : " coals, coke, wood " ; the horse is practically a repetition of her dog formula of 6 ; 0, 3. We see a further step forward in the lines put in as representing the neck between heads and bodies of the two ladies ; the clothes given them

P.C.D.   G

are the same as those which hung in various pictures upon the clothes-line, and are decorated with trimming on the sleeves and hem (Fig. 83).

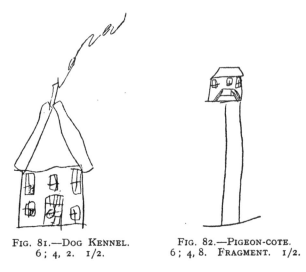

FIG. 81.—DOG KENNEL.   FIG. 82.—PIGEON-COTE.
     6 ; 4, 2.   1/2.   6 ; 4, 8.   FRAGMENT.   1/2.

At 6 ; 5, 2, she drew a series of trees with " leaves " and " berries ", which make a comparatively naturalistic

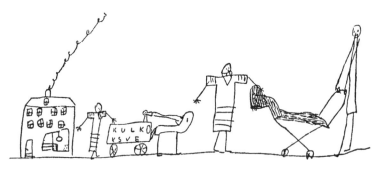

FIG. 83.—A STREET PICTURE.   6 ; 4, 28.   1/2.

impression, although they are really quite formally drawn, with symmetrically arranged, simple branches, and alternately arranged leaves and berries.   In this drawing the influence of the school appears for the first time. She reports that the teacher had drawn such a tree on the blackboard, " Then she rubbed it out, quite quickly, and then we had to draw it." The use of correct localized colour is also to be referred to teaching (Fig. 84, see Plate).

At 6 ; 5, 25, she drew a house and a coal-cart ; a new feature in this picture is seen in the four legs of the horse which for the first time are given in pairs and in outline (Fig. 85).

At 6 ; 6, 1, the picture of a steamship was produced, approaching a landing-stage, upon which a number of persons are seen waiting ; some distance away a man is rowing a boat. The whole situation, the ship with the travellers, the stage with the waiting crowd, is excellently grasped and reproduced, in spite of the formalized representation. Some of the waiting passengers have legs drawn, for the first time, in outline (Fig. 86). In the following period she repeated this drawing several times, once with the ship sinking, and the people saving themselves in a boat.

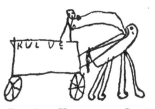

FIG. 85.—HORSE AND CART·
6 ; 5, 25. 1/1.

At Christmas 1924 Margaret made practical use of her art by drawing her Christmas cards herself and giving them to relations and friends. On all of them we see the picture of a Christmas tree, in various forms. One card shows alongside the Christmas tree, several little girls whose faces are in part drawn in profile. These are the first profiles drawn by Margaret, and they likewise resulted from compulsion, for the children had to be looking at the Christmas tree. The profiles are carried out coarsely and inexactly, but do not show the mistake usual with children of mixing a front with a side view. Further, some of the little girls are given hair and strongly marked bows standing straight up into the air on their heads. On the other side stands a little girl : " She is to tell them from Mother, that they are not to dance

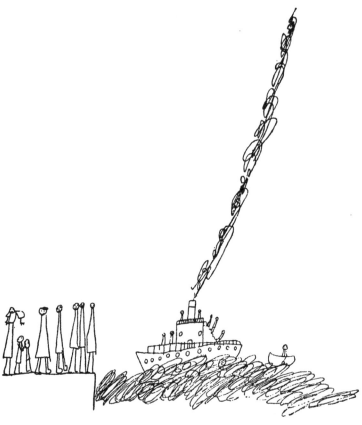

FIG. 86.—A STEAMSHIP APPROACHING THE LANDING-STAGE. 6 ; 6, 1.
1/2.

round the Christmas tree " (at 6 ; 8, 11) (Fig. 87, see Plate facing page 88).

At 6 ; 8, 20, Margaret drew an interior ; " the children " are sitting at table, next to them the servant is standing with a mop, a little farther away " the washerwoman ". In the original there follows, on the same ground line, the scene shown above in the reproduction, namely, " someone shaking a broom so as to spurt water on the tables and chairs ". The wavy scribble appearing on the left was first intended for the wall, but explained as the door. All the figures are carried out in badly executed profile, nose and mouth are represented by the same bend in the line, and the eye is placed at the corner of the mouth. Particular care is taken with the hair

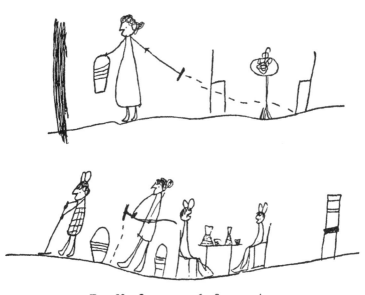

FIG. 88.—INTERIOR. 6 ; 8, 20. 2/3.

and the bow. The handling of the mop is well represented in spite of the primitive single line technique. The round table shows the beginnings of perspective, and the chair is shown in front view with a foreshortened seat (Fig. 88).

At 6 ; 9, 10, a fresh interior was produced, in which the ceilings and walls, table and chair, but not the chest of drawers, are drawn in perspective. The rocking-chair, with a cover thrown over the back, is drawn in a lively

manner, although some lines are missing. The profile
of the woman, with the eye correctly placed, is better

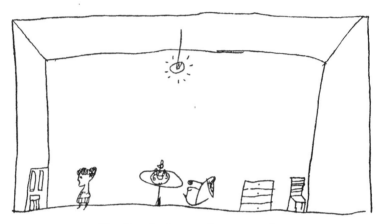

FIG. 89.—INTERIOR.   6 ; 9, 10.   1/2.

worked out than previously. Want of room was given
as the excuse for her head being so much larger than her
body (Fig. 89).

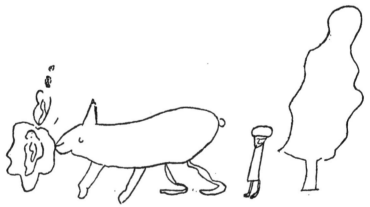

FIG. 90.—HARE EATING CABBAGE.   6 ; 9, 10.   5/6.

On the same day, Margaret drew a hare and " cabbage
that he is eating ".   " Always smaller as they get farther

away," she said, quickly pointing to the cabbages getting smaller towards the top of the drawing. " A tree ", " a boy spying at the hare ". When I remarked that the boy had no arms, I was told : " He's holding them behind his back "—an explanation invented at the moment, since she usually drew her figures without arms.

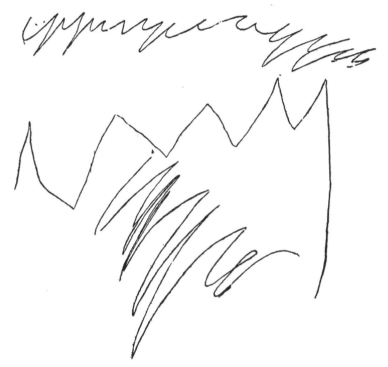

FIG. 91.—SCRIBBLE. 6 ; 9, 10. 2/3.

She complained that the " funny legs " of the hare are so difficult to draw (Fig. 90). The whole is a drawing from memory of a picture in her picture-book. The boy and the tree in the picture-book are at the background, here they are drawn the same size as in the original, but in line with the hare. Concerning the tree she said, as she looked at it afterwards in the picture-book : " That's very difficult to get right, you know. It's so hard to remember it all." Following the winding of the branches of the tree in the book, she once said to herself : " They all go in there." She thus makes the discovery for herself that a complete and accurate memory picture is a necessary condition of getting the drawing right, and for this purpose she tried to impress it on her memory.

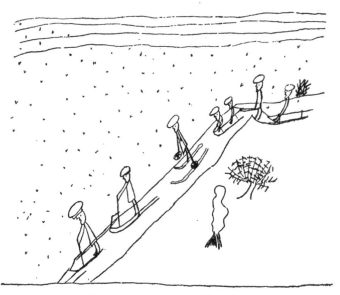

Fig. 92.—Sport Picture. 6 ; 9, 12. The Original sparingly Tinted.

On the same day cursive, zig-zag and wavy scribbling (Fig. 91). A few days later, at 6 ; 9, 12, she drew a sport picture ; children with ski, toboggans, and push-sleighs are running down a hill ; it is snowing, but nevertheless a green tree is standing on the hill, and below it a rather unsuccessful trunk with the outline of branches ; at the top of the picture are " telephone wires ". All figures are in full profile with badly drawn features. The greatest labour has been expended on the ski-caps, which are a novelty in the drawing and hence attracted her attention. For this reason they are also painted in with coloured pencil, while the clothes are not. This motive is often reproduced in the following periods (Fig. 92).

At 6 ; 9, 17, she again drew an interior, a room in perspective ; in it, but not seen from the same point of view, a chair and a table ; the stove forms a new motive in this picture ; the door of the grate is open, and smoke is coming out of it. There is very little colour used (Fig. 93, see Plate).

At 6 ; 9, 24, we have a picture of a " bride " with a wreath and veil and a gigantic bouquet ; the most

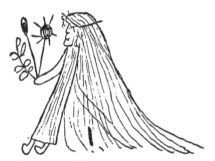

FIG. 94.—A BRIDE.   6 ; 9, 24.   1/1.

notable feature is the soft and life-like line of the arm, which is drawn in outline for the first time. Margaret herself noticed this, for she remarked : " It's really funny that I did the arm so well." Without being asked, she told me how this drawing was produced : " first it was hair " ; the long hair had then reminded her of the veil and in that way the mental picture of a bride occurred to her (Fig. 94). She drew it in outline.

At 6 ; 11, 17, she had been playing at school and made to her scholars an *f* as a copy, the fine lines of which show that her industrious practice of drawing had not been without influence on her writing exercises at school ; also the caricatured *f* which she gave her scholars as a horrible example, is a proof of her sure line (Fig. 95).

The last picture preserved from the end of the seventh year, at about 6 ; 11, is richer in colour, and shows " a girl going to pluck flowers ". The flowers are tulips

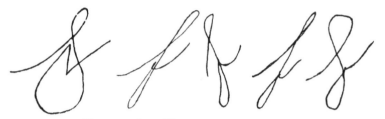

FIG. 95.—COPY WRITING. 6 ; 11, 17. 1/1.

formally drawn, but having, however, in form and colour, a touch of naturalistic representation. A new feature is found in the patterned dress of the girl (Fig. 96, see Plate facing page 82).

THE EIGHTH YEAR

In her eighth year, Margaret's drawings continued for the most part to take the form of composition, but she also frequently drew single objects such as flowers, fruits, utensils ; and liked trying to make them as natural as possible (Figs. 97, 98 ; see Plate facing page 88). At 7 ; 11, 20, she divided up several pages of her drawing-book into squares, and then drew, singly, various objects such as clocks, pictures, basins, umbrellas, brushes, spades, knives, ski, sledges, aeroplanes, caps, gloves, squirrels, anemones, turnips, etc., one in each of the squares ; she also made a number of small compositions, a girl on a sledge, a man in the boat, etc. (Figs. 99, 100 ; see Plate facing page 88). They are all flat pictures.

Particularly towards the end of the year, she made great progress in representing whole figures with their pose and gesture. She drew figures seen from behind, for example, a girl looking at herself in a mirror ; further, figures bending down, for example, a little girl bending over a flower and watering it (Fig. 101, see Plate facing page 88), running figures (Fig. 102 ; age about 7 ; 11, 20 ; see Plate facing page 88).

She probably reached her highest point in this respect at 7 ; 10, 15, with a picture showing a small girl standing on a box : she is bending somewhat forward and handing a flag to a girl standing in front of her ; the folds of the dress in this position are observed and reproduced astonishingly well. The face is seen in semi-profile ; with her other hand she is holding a doll's perambulator, the form of which is drawn with clear and firm lines. The other girl is correspondingly represented with her face directed upwards and her profile turned away, she is bending backwards and stretching out her hands to take hold of the flag. A new feature is the resting position of one leg, the legs being crossed. The pupil of the eye is shown by a blue dot ; the bigger of the two girls has her eye almost behind her ear, and the red of her cheeks at the back of her neck. " Just look what funny hands," remarked Margaret as she looked at the drawing. I asked her why she had drawn them like that. " I couldn't get them out any other way." On the box are " some figures " and the imaginary word " glun ", giving the contents of the box. " As if something was in the box " (Fig. 103, see Plate).

The drawings were often repeated, as was customary with her ; the winter-sport picture done at the end of her seventh year, for example, was repeated every now and then through the whole of her eighth year, although not entirely in a stereotyped fashion. She developed it further, the figures on it became more human, arms and legs received outlines, the clothes were made more complete and carried out entirely in colour. Also in the composition some changes are noticeable. A boy skating is added, sun and blue sky appear instead of the telephone wires. A picture of this kind at 7 ; 8, 17, may be given as an example (Fig. 104, see Plate facing page 90).

As she had already done in her seventh year, she frequently ascribed an imaginary content to her drawings, usually only a short interpretation of the situation ; sometimes she proceeded to make up whole stories with the situation as a starting-point. An example of this is " Karen's Birthday Party " at 7 ; 11, 20. As the drawing of the party is of no great interest in itself, it is not reproduced here. Of the twenty-five little girls who are Karen's guests, some are sitting at a long table with their backs to the beholder, with cups of chocolate and plates of cake in front of them (Fig. 105). On the other side of the table is a row of girls drawn in profile, one standing with her back turned and looking out of the green-curtained window; at the end of the table we have Karen, who, being the most important person, is half as large again as the others ; at the

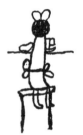

FIG. 105. — FROM " KAREN'S BIRTH-DAY PARTY ". FRAG-MENT. ABOUT 7; 11, 20. ORIGINAL IN COLOURS. 1/1.

side, five or six little girls are standing before the green curtain, and the attempt at natural grouping is evident ; some have their backs turned, two are in profile, one is facing the beholder, and one can only be seen with difficulty at the back. Three have their arms affectionately entwined, on the other side there are two or three little girls round a lady with a perambulator. The character of the corresponding story which was, by way of exception, written down, may be seen from the following fragment.

KAREN'S BIRTHDAY PARTY

" Karen : good-day to all twenty-five guests. Marianne : congratulate you Karen, here is a parcel. Ruth : now we will play ' last man out ', won't we ? yes we will said Karen . . . Marianne : Elli has it, look out Björg, don't go too near. Björg : you've got it Marianne. Elli thinks of nothing, stands on both legs as Marianne comes running up and says Elli you've got it. Elli : no I haven't. You haven't surely. Elli : we'll play something else. Elli : can't we play hide-and-seek. Let's play hide-and-seek says Karen, yes say all the guests, let's play hide-and-seek," etc.

The style is as formalized as the drawing, but is a fairly faithful representation of little girls playing together.

The motives in themselves often come from her imagination and are made into fairy-story pictures. This is true of a drawing of a witch stirring her witches' cauldron, at 8 ; o, 8. " A little girl has come to the witch, and now she is to be set free." A drawing, at about 7 ; 10, 15, represents two Court ladies, each sitting on a chair with a kind of sceptre in her hand ; Margaret explains these as " rods ", which they move towards one another when they are talking. In the doorway stands the Queen, who has just entered. On the original drawing the clothes are in colour ; the attempt to draw correctly the legs of the figures sitting down is noteworthy. As we are in a castle, the decoration is richer than usual, the chairs are decorated with knobs, windows and doors with round arches, and the tiny figures on the door frame are there " to make it grand " (Fig. 106).

Her childish imagination was also very active when drawing the airship *Norge*, at 8 ; o, 11. We see two figures who, as Margaret explained, " have put on wings and are going to fly away ". The modern marvel of the airship has thus awakened the idea of primitive human attempts to fly, as in the ancient legend of Icarus. The wings are drawn both from the front and in profile fairly correctly. The conception of the *Norge* floating over the roofs of the houses is expressed in the nature of the terrain, which is made a hill, half of the upper house disappearing beneath the line of vision given by

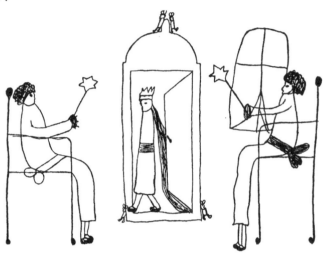

FIG. 106.—TWO COURT LADIES AND THE QUEEN. ABOUT 7 ; 10, 15.
ORIGINAL IN COLOURS. 1/2.

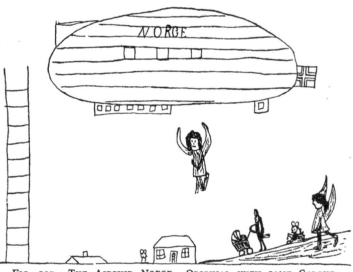

FIG. 107.—THE AIRSHIP *NORGE*. ORIGINAL WITH SOME COLOUR.
8 ; 0, 11. 1/2.

the edge of the paper, while of the lower house only the
roof is seen ; in the same way only the head of a figure
at the bottom of the hill is visible.   On the left is a
ladder for climbing up to the airship.   The drawing has
only a small amount of colour, the hill is green, the roof
red, and the Norwegian flag is given in the correct colours
(Fig. 107).

We have already seen that caricature can occur in
very early children's drawings.   Her drawing at 8 ; 0, 10,

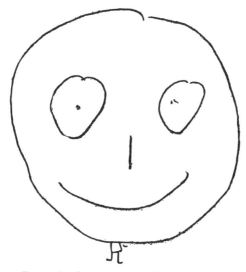

FIG. 108.—CARICATURES.   8 ; 0, 10.   1/2.

shows a tremendous disproportion between head and
body, perhaps also the shape of the line representing
the mouth was done on purpose ; further, the drawing
is done in a primitive style which she had otherwise
long ago abandoned (Fig. 108).

Now and then attempts at ornamental drawing appear
(see page 176).   As showing that even in the eighth year
scribbling still occurred, we may note a wavy scribble
of the most primitive description carried out in green
pencil at 7 ; 11, 20 (Fig. 109).

In the eighth year *colour* was the main new development. Margaret now carried almost all her drawings out in colour, she preferred coloured pencils, but also used water-colours. We are not able to give many of these drawings on account of the cost of reproducing them, hence, apart from the sport picture and the girl with the flag, I only give three from the end of the year (at about 7 ; 10, 15). From these we can best see how Margaret's development in drawing had advanced up to her eighth year.

The drawing at the top left hand of the first picture (Fig. 110, see Plate facing this page) represents her father and a friend of his playing chess. The two round table

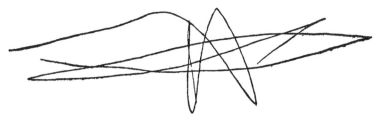

FIG. 109.—SCRIBBLE.   7 ; 11, 20.   2/3.

tops are given in correct perspective, as is the chess-board. The latter, however, is from another view-point, appearing as a rhombus instead of a trapeze. The next picture shows two little girls fairly correctly drawn at a table; there is here no overlapping or transparency, but the perspective of the table is once more given from another point of view than that of the chairs. The small table next to it is supposed to represent a writing-table with a telephone. She doubtless wanted to put it in the background, but it appears on the same line with the dining-table. A little girl is standing with her back turned at the extreme right at the water-tap, raising her arms and turning both taps at once ; the drawing exhibits an accomplishment which she had only just acquired, namely that of representing figures from behind, the movement being likewise well given. The lower picture represents the interior of a bedroom, which is proof of her power of correct and harmonious representation. The mother and the little girl form a natural group, and the manner in which the mother is doing the child's hair with the hair ribbon slung over her hand, is very accurately observed. On the left, the child's cot is fairly correctly drawn ; the most notable part of the drawing is the perspective of the door leading into the other room ; but here again the panels of the door are drawn as lop-sided rectangles instead of trapezes.

The second picture (Fig. 111, see Plate facing page 98), which is a part of St. Hanshaugen, was drawn from memory. It immediately gives the impression of a life-like and comparatively correct picture showing the path at the side of the harbour, the tower, the grass slope, the flight of steps, the path with seats, and a little girl with a perambulator, all seen however from an almost impossible point of view, namely, a point on a level with the upper limit of the grass slope. The walking figures are quite well worked out, apart from their badly executed facial profiles, and their hands which are stuck somewhat too far forward. The flight of steps and the grass slope connect the two surfaces in a natural manner. The whole composition produces a harmonious and natural effect. The sky is blue, but the weather signals on the tower foretell bad weather, probably because these particular signals make the best effect on the drawing. This motive also had been drawn several times previously. The rapidity of Margaret's progress in the immediately preceding time is best seen by comparing this drawing with her picture of St. Hanshaugen of a year and a half previously, at 6 ; 3, 1.

The third picture (Fig. 112, see Plate facing page 98) represents a house with a garden, figures, etc. The same subject had been drawn countless times before in the most various forms, but this one is unusually rich and carefully done. The house is drawn, as always from the beginning of her eighth year, with a gable, but without any attempt at linear perspective ; on the other hand, the open door is drawn in perspective, but only the lower line is correct, the upper one should have run in the opposite direction. The mistake arises from the fact that she had previously correctly given the perspective of doors opening inwards by showing the lines sloping together towards one another, and in this case, when the door opens outwards, she is unable quite to free herself from the preconception. The drawing shows very good power of expressing pose and movement ; we see this in the case of the girl in the half-open door, holding with one hand on to the door-post and gripping the door-latch with the other, in the walking movements of the pedestrians, in the slope of the flag waving on the flag-staff, but above all in the surprisingly natural drawing of the little girl who has thrown herself on the ground at the corner of the house, " in order to smell the flowers ". She is resting on her hands, her body has a characteristic steep curve upwards, her toes are pressed into the earth, her yellow hair is flying in the wind. The picture order is harmonious. There is no background, no horizon.

Among the pedestrians we recognize again the pair seen in the picture of St. Hanshaugen, but this time they have important-looking brown leather suitcases in their hands, which are stretched somewhat too far forward. These figures, either separately or together, had been appearing in Margaret's drawing for some time previously. The man carries a stick or a handbag, he may or may not have a pipe. Sometimes also he appears, full of youth and spirit, on a sport picture with a push-sleigh. The lady has a bag or a suitcase, or she is pushing a perambulator. She may also be skating, and then appears in a brightly coloured sporting dress with a wide skirt, but can still be recognized by her head-gear. Or she is standing on the pier at the steamer " Stavanger-fjord ", and has just put down her huge trunk in order to remove, with a large pocket-handkerchief, the tears of pain, visibly dropping from her eyes, and caused by her having to leave her beloved Fatherland.

The red toy balloons show that this drawing was made during the month of the Spring sales ; the idea, that the little girl with the perambulator is coming direct out of a large city stores, has little connection with the countrified look of the house and its surroundings, but on an imaginary picture everything is allowed. Hence the imagination has been allowed to play with the colours —the curtains shimmer with rainbow colour, produced by a curious point-technique, and the roof is green ; Margaret explains that it is a peat roof, and when asked why she drew a peat roof, said that it was prettier than a red roof. This same pleasure in colour characterizes the whole drawing, as Margaret's other drawings in the last year. When, for example, she gives her ladies and little girls long hair and ribbons, often tied into large bows, in complete contradiction to the fashion of the time, she certainly only does this because it allows her to go in for a greater richness in line and colour. The broad grass slope and the long row of flowers on the wall of the house add to the general impression of brilliant colour. The blue sky is a wavy scribble, the sun a circular scribble, wherein we may see relationships between these last drawings of hers and her first.

Before closing this report of Margaret's development in drawing, I ought to attempt to answer the question whether it may be regarded as typical of children in general, or whether Margaret had an unusually developed talent for drawing. I think I may say her talent was not above the average, but this was not true of the interest that she felt for drawing. But if we ask whether children of the same age are in general as far advanced as Margaret, the answer is certainly in the negative. The usual mistakes in children's drawings, such as transparency, overlapping, etc., hardly appeared in her drawings at all ; in respect of perspective and composition, and perhaps also in the matter of lifelike and natural expression, she was without doubt in advance of her age.   But her drawings never lost the typical formalized stamp of children's drawings, and they never show signs of the sensitive working out of outline and detail, which is perhaps the surest characteristic of artistic endowment in children.   Hence I would like to take it as fundamental in judging her drawing, that its development was typically childlike, but that in many respects she was more advanced than the majority of children of the same age.

GENERAL VIEW OF THE DEVELOPMENT AND PSYCHOLOGY OF CHILDREN'S DRAWINGS

THE study of the early drawing of children shows that a significant and regulated development is found in the apparently valueless and planless drawing of children. It appears on the one hand as a progress in ability to draw and in increasing mastery of line and form ; on the other hand, progress in drawing is the expression of the gradual unfolding of the child's soul. For drawing is, like talking, a means of expression, crippled and undeveloped in the case of most grown-up people, but in the case of children still alive and full of activity, however incomplete the products may appear to adult eyes.

If now we start from the steps in development of children's drawings which have been recognized as existent, we find that Margaret's drawings belong mainly to the two first steps : the period of scribbling and that of formula ; but that in the latter years many characteristics of the two following upper stages are revealed: the stage of the flat picture with formal traits and the stage of line plastic pictures, perspective drawing and line space pictures.

SCRIBBLING

Under the word scribbling I understand all free drawing of lines having no representative or decorative purpose.

Investigation of Margaret's drawing shows that there were several distinctly recognizable steps in the development of her scribbling : (1) Wavy scribbling, (2) Circular scribbling, (3) Variegated scribbling, to which belongs the scribbling of zig-zag lines, straight lines, angles, crosses, ovals, spirals, loops, rectangles, wavy lines, imitation of handwriting, etc. As regards the placing of the scribble upon paper, here again we are able to distinguish three successive stages in the first early drawings. 1. Mass scribble : the scribble is placed in the middle of the paper in dense masses. 2. Scattered scribble : the scribbles are made with larger spaces between the lines and scattered over the whole surface of the paper, certain line formations, obviously belonging together, appearing more plainly. 3. Isolated scribble : single lines and forms are drawn and repeated separately.

Wavy and circular scribble have also been recognized as the first steps by other investigators, for example Major,[1] Dix [2] and Krötzsch.[3] Whether the other phases which I have observed are also found in the drawings of other children on more exact observation, is, for the present, an open question. The observations of most biographers are not devoted to the very earliest beginnings of the development of drawing, but usually commence with the first clear, isolated form produced by the child, and hence are not exhaustive enough to decide this question.

How does scribbling come about, and what is its meaning regarded as drawing, and from the psychological point of view ?

The child begins to scribble because it sees grown-up people and other children drawing or writing and wishes to do the same. But it is by no means impossible that children who come into possession of the necessary materials would commence to draw on their own initiative. We have to suppose that, apart from the tendency to imitation, other circumstances might play a part, for example inherited aptitude for graphical expression, and inborn tendencies in the brain, muscles, and mental constitution. It is true that the tendency to imitation is alone sufficient to explain the child's commencing to draw, but it does not explain the interest and the per-

[1] loc. cit., pp. 46 et seq.   [2] loc. cit., p. 70.   [3] loc. cit., pp. 7, 9.

sistence with which the child continues its drawing for months and years without external stimulation or request. Scribbling has also an affective element ; the child takes delight in the monotonous play of lines and movement, and this feeling applies both to the sense impressions and to the movement. It feels pleasure in seeing and feeling the movements in the hand, and in observing the line appearing on the paper, exactly in the same way as children, from the middle of the first year, take a pleasure in watching, touching, and handling objects. Finally, scribbling is also the result of the desire of the child for occupation, and of its natural drive towards movement and action.

Some investigators, such as Bühler, regard the first scribbling exclusively as a game of movement, and assert that the child is at first only imitating the movements of the hand, frequently without realizing its connection with the lines which result on the paper.[1] This is wrong according to my observations ; Margaret's attention was already attracted by the very first lines. She looked at them with obvious interest, and seeing them appear clearly gave her pleasure.

Nevertheless, the first scribbling is chiefly associated with movement, and its production directly dependent upon this. This is mainly true of the two first stages— wavy scribble and circular scribble—and here again particularly of wavy scribble. This is produced by the hand which holds the pencil moving to-and-fro in a free pendulum-like motion from the elbow or shoulder-joint ; in this way wavy scribble is produced quite involuntarily, without any need for the child's will being involved, in the form of slightly curved lines. Generally speaking, the hand is moved quite gradually downwards on the paper during the scribbling, so that each following arc is produced directly under the one before, otherwise the later lines would coincide with the first and not be visible. In this progressive motion, as well as in the

[1] *loc. cit.*, p. 133.

first start and at each turn at the end-points, a certain activity of the child's will must exist, but otherwise wavy scribble is essentially mechanical, with but a very small psychical element. If the arm lies straight on the paper, the swings are horizontal, if the arm is horizontal they are vertical, while a diagonal position produces diagonal lines.   Psychically speaking, wavy scribble has the object of laying, by practice, the first foundation of the relationship between the impulse to draw, innervation of the brain, the muscular movement mechanism, and the eye's power to apprehend the line; and also the practice of each of these separately. The gently curved form is advantageous, as the eye can follow it more easily than the straight line.   This first foundation of drawing, if begun at an early age, must be practised for several months before it is firmly enough inculcated for the child to take the next step to circular scribble. Wavy scribbling is the fundamental form of all drawing, the primitive cell from which all graphic art grows.

Although wavy scribble is the typical exercise of the first period, it is not the only one. Now and then we have the scribbling of shorter lines appearing more by chance and in various directions, and of isolated angles, loops, points but never of distinct rounded forms.

Circular scribbling shows a higher stage of development, for the child, in order to be able to produce circular forms, has to make more conscious hand movement. But the movement necessary for circular scribbling is also simple and mechanical, for the hand is simply led round in a circle uniformly and repeatedly.   This movement also can be made freely from the shoulder or elbow, but is transferred more and more to the wrist and fingers as practice progresses.

From this point circular scribbling, now and then interrupted by wavy scribble and other casually reproduced scribbling of lines, forms for some time the main type of exercise ; but as soon as the graphic movements connected with it have acquired surety, variously formed scribble is produced. This consists, as already remarked, of zig-zag lines, angles, crosses, straight lines, and other simple lines and forms. At the same time the scribble is scattered over the paper. This kind of scribble requires shorter, more differentiated, and better adapted movements (particularly of wrist and finger), a greater capacity for apprehending, distinguishing and separating lines and forms from one another, more numerous mental pictures, better memory, greater combination of will-impulses, more practised and orderly arrangement of imagination and movement, more flexible motor mechanism. Altogether, it makes considerably greater demand on mental development than wavy and circular scribbling, which are more mechanical in their nature. From the point of view of drawing it means that the child acquires a store of elementary lines and forms, which are brought into service for representative drawing later on.

Pure scribbling is a planless and expressionless drawing, which is carried out without a definite purpose, and in no way expresses the child's imaginings; it is a stage preliminary to that of actual drawing. It is a definitely ideomotor process agreeing with the well-known law, that the mental picture of a movement is the beginning of the movement itself. It is a process moving in a circle and mechanically repeated, showing little signs of progress; in other words, distinctly a process of practice. For purposes of practice, scribbling still maintains its place even when the child has already passed on to representative drawing; new forms, such as rectangles, the forms of handwriting, and lines and forms already learned, such as zig-zag lines, spirals, etc., are practised and mastered by repeated scribbling. This at any rate was the case with Margaret. As long as I observed her drawing, that is into the last months of the eighth year, scribbling still continued to occur. Also in the case of another little girl, age 4 ; 3, I noticed scribbling alongside fairly well developed formalized drawing. Whether this is also usual in the case of children, I have not been able to discover from other biographical studies on children's drawings. These almost imply that scribbling ceased with the transition to formalized drawing; but this can hardly agree with the actual facts.

THE TRANSITION FROM SCRIBBLING TO FORMALIZED DRAWING

Whilst still at the stage which I have called variegated scribbling, Margaret began to repeat consciously certain formations of lines which had been produced by chance. Among these particularly noticeable was a small dense zig-zag scribble with a long line which was repeated again and again in much the same form. She also began to ascribe to this and other chance groups of lines a name: "It's Mama", "It's a flag"; shortly afterwards she began to announce her intention beforehand: "Draw Mama", "Draw flag". From this point onward the scribbled groups of lines must be given the value of a symbolic representation of real things, and this symbolic scribbling now forms the transition to intelligible drawing.

Other investigators, who have made similar observations, for example, Major and Bühler, have maintained that the child, when it gives its scribbled lines a name, means nothing but the game of scribbling in itself; in giving names in this way it is merely chattering in imitation of grown-up people. They maintain that there is in no sense any representative intention, that no picture of the thing is seen by the inner eye of the child, and that its imagination does not cheat it into seeing a likeness of the real thing.[1] Major thinks that the child's imagination is not yet powerful enough to allow him to see something real in his scribble.[2]

My observations tell me that the child actually intends to represent something; for this was plainly

---

[1] Bühler, *loc. cit.*, pp. 133, 134.
[2] Major, *loc. cit.*, pp. 51 *et seq.*

announced by Margaret when she said " Draw Mama " ; why indeed should not the imagination of a child be able to cheat it into the belief that a line is a human being, when it makes the child believe, after all, that a piece of wood is a doll, or a stick a horse ? Some of Margaret's scribbled groups of lines, for example, the small zig-zag line ending in the longer stroke, might possibly be said to actually recall a head and a body, or a flag and the flagstaff ; it is true of course that this form could not, without powerful assistance of the child's imagination, appear to have the slightest likeness to the " floor ", the " mirror ", or the " dress ".

Margaret's next step in the direction of the human formula consists in a double circular scribble, isolated and repeated in the same form, this being designated " Mama ". We may surely suppose that this round form reminded her of a head, which is for a child the most noticeable part of the human form.[1] This supposition is all the more justified by the fact that she reverted to representing human beings by a scribble again and again in the following years, even up to 2 ; 7.

The proof that her attention remained attached to the circular form and its value as a means of representation is further given by the fact that she continued to practise rounded forms together with straight lines and loops ; and it is these exercises in the form of isolated scribble which lead in a short time to the first primitive formalized human form usual with children : a circle with two straight lines—called " Mama ".

This agrees with Bühler's description : " Mental progress towards intelligible drawing may, like that from babbling to intelligible speech, take place in two somewhat distinct ways, either namely, by the child discovering a known form in its own lines and being thereby stimulated to repeat them, or by its having learned the practice of making pictures by watching

---

[1] Cf. Sully, *loc. cit.*, p. 333 ; Levinstein, *Kinderzeichnungen bis zum 14. Lebensjahr*, p. 5.

others, and then attempting one day to do the same itself. These matters deserve a greater interest than they have hitherto found, for they are examples of the few earliest discoveries made by the child in its mental life, and can easily be followed objectively." [1] In Margaret's case we have to reckon with both ways, for something was drawn almost daily for her amusement, at her own request. On the other hand, my observations do not agree with Bühler's further remark: "When once this step has been taken, its general effect quickly appears, either immediately after the first case, or in any case after a few repetitions; the effect is similar to that when we grown-up people have suddenly become possessed of a piece of new general knowledge. In every case henceforward, when the child makes lines in play it brings to its game the right attitude, namely the intention to represent something." [2] In the case of Margaret's drawing no general effect appeared; the tendency to scribble continued into her eighth year, alongside representative drawing, although to a diminishing degree. My observations also give me no confirmation for the following further remarks: "A child does not usually grasp quite as quickly the fact that the most various objects can be represented graphically, and often remains for a considerable time at the few objects concerning which it made its discovery. That is to say, drawing still means the same for it as the construction of one of its figures and hence also frequently gets quite a special name, for example, ' make man ', or other such names." [3] Margaret was already aware at her first transitional period, that the most various things could be drawn; she had seen them drawn by other people and she even herself proposed things which she had never seen drawn: " draw floor ", " draw mirror ". The fact that the child limits itself to a few objects is no doubt mainly due to the good reason that

---

[1] Bühler, *loc. cit.*, pp. 135, 136.
[2] *loc. cit.*, p. 136.　　　[3] *loc. cit.*, p. 136.

technical difficulties prohibit it from attempting others. According to Lukens' conclusion there is a transitional stage between scribbling and formalized drawing, which he calls the period of local arrangement. The child makes use of groups of scribbled lines, arranging them in fairly correct relation to one another to stand for the most various things which it desires to represent. For example, a scribble is to represent the head, a couple of other scribbled lines a long way below, the legs of a human being.[1] I could not detect anything resembling this localized arrangement in Margaret's drawing, and I have found no confirmation of it in other biographical studies, unless perhaps Bubi's drawings of a cart may be taken in this sense.[2]

FORMALIZED DRAWING

The child's first drawing is usually a formalized[3] human figure ; but it has also been reported that children here and there have begun with animals or other things. The first human formula is very primitive, and only grasped with great uncertainty by the child. Margaret repeated it several times, and then it was forgotten again ; a new one was developed, but this degenerated in a short time to a round scribble, and even the third was not permanent ; it was only at the beginning of

[1] Lukens, *A Study of Children's Drawing in the Early Years*, pp. 80, 81.

[2] Scupin, *loc. cit.*, pp. 166, 262.

[3] [Certain terms in this book were the subject of some thought and discussion on the part of Dr. Eng, the editor, and myself, as regards the most suitable English equivalents. I used " formula ", " formalized ", etc., for the German *Schema*, etc. Dr. Eng pointed out that, although " schema ", " schematized ", etc., are very rarely used in English, some English psychologists have adopted them. She cites Judd (*Psychology of Secondary Education*), Goodenough (*Measurement of Intelligence by Drawing*), Wooster Curti (*Child Psychology*).

In spite of this, it was decided to use " formula ", etc., as these terms are already in common use in the same sense in connection with drawing and painting generally. It seems unnecessary to introduce a new term, which has the grave disadvantage of being closely similar to a common word, " scheme ", having an allied meaning.

Schwingkritzeln is translated by " wavy scribbling ", as its nature is fully discussed in the text. " Swing scribbling " would be the nearest equivalent.—*Trans.*]

her fifth year that her representation of the human figure became a firmly fixed element in her drawing. Details, such as eyes and fingers, fared similarly. This course of events is quite analogous in observations made concerning the development of the child's concepts. For example, some observers report that the first expression for " I " disappears again, and only appears again after several months ; numerical concepts may be correctly grasped and made use of, only to disappear shortly afterwards and not to be re-acquired with certainty for a very considerable time.[1] Altogether, the first concepts of a child are quite generally characterized by great uncertainty, and this also appears to be the fate of the first formalized drawing. The first drawings of human beings made by a child usually consist of structures having only heads and legs (*Kopffüssler*, *têtard*), and these are very gradually made more complete. As Luquet has shown, *têtard*-figures also frequently occur in primitive savage art.[2] Even in her sixth year, Margaret still drew human beings without a neck or hair, often even without arms. Lena Partridge gives an account of an investigation showing how many children at each age include in their drawings the most important details.

Year :	4.	5.	6.	7.	8.	9.	10.	11.	12.	13.
	%	%	%	%	%	%	%	%	%	%
Body- -	50	82	92	93	98	99	98	99	100	100
Legs - -	39	83	92	93	94	98	98	97	98	98
Arms -	45	67	71	80	76	85	93	90	95	95
Neck - -	8	22	20	37	51	63	79	79	90	93
Hair - -	6	26	27	32	38	58	70	65	73	82
Clothing-	16	29	42	56	63	77	82	91	93	99
Hat - -	32	57	59	76	78	81	84	89	85	80
Buttons -	30	37	37	52	55	66	64	81	79	83 [3]

The child at first always draws its human beings full face, then gradually passes on to the representation of

[1] Cf. Helga Eng, *Abstrakte Begriffe im Sprechen und Denken des Kindes*, Leipzig, 1914, p. 4.

[2] G.-H. Luquet, " Les bonhommes têtard dans le dessin enfantin ". *Journal de Psychologie*, 17, pp. 692 *et seq.*

[3] Lena Partridge, *loc. cit.*, pp. 166 *et seq.*

profile, but not in such a way as to suddenly produce its figures in full profile. On the contrary, single parts of the body are turned sideways at different times, in an order which is given by Lena Partridge as follows : first the feet, then the nose, then eyes and mouth, then the arms, and finally the body.[1] Krötzsch gives the order : feet, arms, head, body.[2] Margaret's order was : feet, arms, body, head ; the fact that she drew the body in profile at a comparatively early period was due to her attempting to represent seated figures. It is thus that mixed drawings are produced, having some parts in profile and others full face. One may often observe children drawing the nose in profile but adding two eyes, frequently the mouth, and sometimes even a second nose full face (Fig. 113). About one-half of all profile drawings between the sixth and the ninth year show this mixture, and according to Lena Partridge, it is rare to come across a perfectly executed profile representation even into the thirteenth year, although the tendency to profile drawing becomes from year to year stronger during the school age.[3]

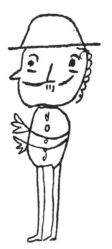

FIG. 113.—MIXED PROFILE. (FROM RICCI.) 1/1.

First the head only is drawn in outline, then follow the body, the legs, and finally the arms. According to Lena Partridge, at the age of seven only 42 per cent of the arms are in outline, but 88 per cent of the legs.[4] Margaret was still drawing arms and legs as simple lines in her seventh year ; at 6 ; 6, 1, the legs were outlined for the first time, and at 6 ; 9, 24, the arms.

In order to represent the details of the human form,

[1] loc. cit., pp. 169, 170.   [2] loc. cit., p. 80.
[3] loc. cit., p. 170.   [4] loc. cit., p. 168.

the child uses a somewhat different technique and form at various periods, but usually there is progressive development.

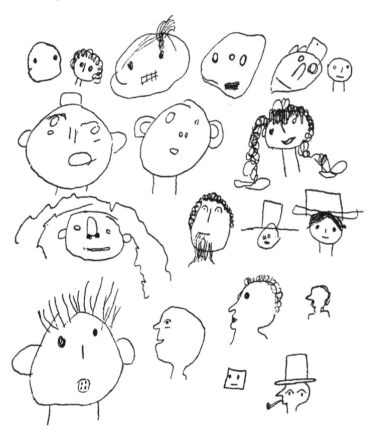

FIG. 114.—HEADS: DRAWN BY BEGINNERS (GIRLS 6; 3, to 8; 3) IN THE ELEMENTARY SCHOOL AT OSLO. THE TWO LAST FROM RICCI. 5/6.

The head is generally shown as a circle, sometimes as an oval, but rarely as a rectangle (Fig. 114). Of the features, the eyes receive the child's main attention, they are drawn in the earliest and rarely forgotten;

the mouth is sometimes, and the nose frequently omitted, as in the full-face view it does not play so important a part. The eyes are points, circles, points surrounded by circles; later on the eyelids or eyebrows are shown by curved lines.

The nose appears as a circle, straight line, oval, triangle, rectangle, cross, open angle, narrow rectangle, crooked line, and later on in profile; the mouth as a line going straight across the whole circle of the face, as two parallel lines, as an oval, rarely as a circle, but it may also be given as a rectangle or spindle-shaped. The teeth are points, straight lines, zig-zag lines; the ears, which are not drawn so frequently, are rounded figures standing out from each side of the head, in the profile they are often given as ovals, but sometimes more true to nature. The hair is shown by lines, zig-zags, or spirals. The neck, long neglected, is finally shown as a straight stroke or a rectangle, between head and body; it is only later that it is produced along with the head and the body in a continuous line. The body is at first only the open space between two lines which represent both body and legs; later on, it is marked off by a cross-stroke and also represented by an oval, a circle, or a rectangle; the attempt is finally made to make it more naturalistic (Fig. 115). The legs are seen as simple lines, and later in outline; the feet are simple lines at right angles to the line of the legs, or oval or circular in shape, as loops, as rectangles, and finally truer to nature, with the outline of the feet or boots (Fig. 116). The arms are straight lines sloping downwards and outwards, often horizontal and sometimes stretched upwards, last of all they are placed in the natural position hanging down at the sides; they are frequently joined to the head or placed too far down on the body. The fingers are drawn as a loose bundle of lines or as cross-strokes added to the arm line; the hand is given as a cross-line at the end of the arm-line, and under this cross-line the fingers are added like the teeth of a rake; or the fingers are spread out in all directions. Later on, the hand is made into a circle or an oval and the fingers are given an out-

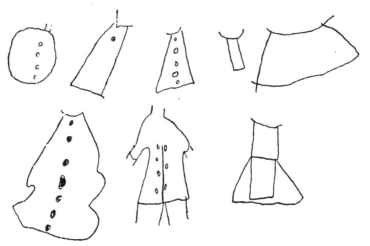

FIG. 115.—BODIES. DRAWN BY BEGINNERS AT THE ELEMENTARY SCHOOL IN OSLO. 10/11.

line or else in a line. Finally, both hand and fingers are drawn in a single outline, and then frequently in

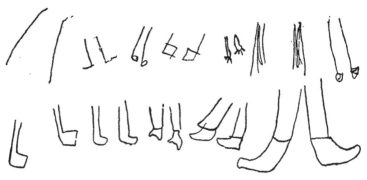

FIG. 116.—LEGS. DRAWN BY BEGINNERS AT THE ELEMENTARY SCHOOL IN OSLO. ABOUT 5/6.

a small ragged shape ; sometimes, also, the hand and particularly the hand grasping an object is given as a circular scribble. The fingers are often too many or too few, but later the definite number five is produced (Fig. 117).[1]

Next to the representation of human beings, animals are preferred in children's drawings, according to the observations of several investigators, as they are lively and mobile creatures which attract the child's attention to a high degree.[2] In Margaret's drawing they are very rarely taken as a model, and this also appears to me to be the case in the drawings of other children. In a beginners' class of seven-year-old little girls, during

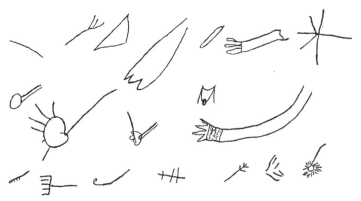

FIG. 117.—ARMS AND HANDS DRAWN BY BEGINNERS AT THE ELEMEN-TARY SCHOOL IN OSLO. THE LOWEST ROW FROM SULLY. ABOUT 5/6.

the first few days, before school had been able to influence the ability to draw, I gave a number of exercises in free drawing from memory ; these consisted in the representation of a man, a house, an apple, a carrot, and a horse. Finally, they were then to make another drawing of a subject chosen by themselves. In the case of this free choice of subject, the four first-named subjects were repeated by a great many, but only one girl chose the horse for repetition ; also, with the exception of a

[1] Cf. Sully, Levinstein, Ricci, and others.
[2] Stern, *Psychologie der frühen Kindheit*, p. 242 ; Bühler, *loc. cit.*, p. 141 ; Levinstein, *loc. cit.*, p. 17.

single case of a bird, no other animals were chosen for representation. This must be interpreted as showing that the children were not particularly interested in the animal subject, and did not feel capable of mastering it.

Louise Maitland found from the examination of 1,570 free drawings of school children, that 33 per cent drew human beings, 25 per cent houses, 41 per cent utensils and other things from their daily life, 27 per cent plants, while only 18 per cent attempted animals. At the age of five to ten years, about a quarter of the children drew animals, and those between eleven and seventeen only a tenth.[1] Katzaroff came to similar conclusions.[2]

Domestic animals are particularly beloved in children's drawings, and of these again, the four-legged ; later on, birds, and more rarely fish, butterflies and others are represented.

When animals occur in the earliest attempts at drawing, they have to pass through a similar period of development to that which is found in the case of the human figure. A circular scribble alone, or in connection with several lines representing legs, is a dog, a horse, etc. ; this may also be shown in the form of a general outline of an animal body, which is not much more than an uncertain outlining of a surface. Here, also, development proceeds to a more or less correct formalized drawing.

Children often begin drawing animals when they have already acquired a formula for the human figure. This is then often made use of to represent the animal, by simply placing the body horizontally and giving it four legs and a tail, the human face remaining unaltered (Fig. 118).

When children have learned some kind of animal form, they make use of it to represent the most various

[1] Louise Maitland, *What Children draw to Please Themselves*, p. 87, quoted from E. Barnes, " Children's Drawings ", III, *Studies in Education*, 2, p. 109.

[2] Katzaroff, "Qu'est-ce que les enfants dessinent ? " *Archives de Psychologie*, 9, pp. 125–133.

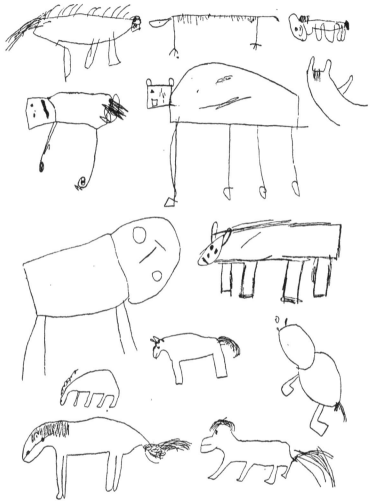

FIG. 118.—THE HORSE. DRAWN BY BEGINNERS AT THE ELEMENTARY SCHOOL IN OSLO. 1/2.

species of animals, by adding to it small details corresponding to the most important characteristic features. Levinstein reports concerning his experiments in drawing, that a bird formula was turned into a dog merely by adding a second pair of legs, or into a fish by the removal of all legs ; conversely a bird is produced from a dog by two legs being removed. The child also frequently forgets to make the most necessary alterations. A little girl of eight years of age drew, on the roof of a house, a four-legged animal with long ears and said that it was a " swallow ". When someone said that it must surely be a dog, she laughed at him and said " dogs don't sit on the roof ".[1] " A flower," " a tree " are also formulæ in children's drawing which are made use of for all sorts of flowers and trees, and we meet the same trait in the drawing of houses, ships, etc.

This method of repetition and minor alteration is said to be predominant in the work and art of primitive races : " When a savage makes a weapon, he modifies or copies a weapon ; when he makes a vessel he modifies or copies a vessel." [2]   The circumstance, that the child makes use of the same formula for many and various animals, has its parallels in the development of the child's concepts. When the child is learning to speak, the various animals are at first described by the same word. Margaret, for example, uses " bow-wow ", for dog, cat, bear, wolf, fox, horse, etc. These first, all-inclusive concepts of the child have been called primary concepts, In the same way, we might designate its much too comprehensive formula as the primary formula.

The primary formulæ of the child become gradually differentiated in the same way as do the primary concepts : it no longer uses the same formula to represent human beings, four-legged animals, birds, and fishes, but instead produces a fairly acceptable formula for each species. Differentiation advances, the child no longer uses the same formula for all four-legged animals, but now proceeds to show approximately the real appearance of the dog, the horse, etc., so that one is able to decide from the drawing what animal is meant.

---

[1] Levinstein, *loc. cit.*, p. 21.
[2] W. H. Holmes, quoted from Chamberlain, *The Child*, p. 197.

The most ancient folk art begins, like that of the child, with animal drawings of an undifferentiated formalized character.[1]

While the child always draws human beings full face at first, animals are shown sideways from the very beginning, for the characteristic appearance of an animal is best seen from the profile view. At first, for example, the dog gets a large number of legs, but a child learns comparatively quickly to grasp and represent the four legs correctly, this being made easier by the fact that they belong together in pairs. But this very fact is not always shown in the drawing, for often the four legs are put on at equal intervals. Many children also draw only two legs, as they think that "you can't see those on the other side". In the earliest palæolithic art also (the art of the older Stone Age), animals are drawn in "absolute profile", with only two legs, and frequently also with equal spacings between all four legs drawn very primitively ; the legs, as in children's drawings, often having no feet, and are frequently incomplete or entirely missing.[2]

At first, the body is often drawn to begin with, then the head, legs, and tail ; or head and body are drawn in a single outline together, and the other parts added. It is only at a later stage that the whole outline is drawn in one stroke. The body is also frequently drawn as a single straight line. The covering of hair is often drawn standing out like a halo of strokes from the line of the back, or around the whole outline. The child's animal drawings are in general better proportioned than its human drawings, perhaps because the child only begins to devote itself to them at a later stage of development.

In the matter of trees, the child has definite formulæ, which suggest the chief characteristic of the tree, trunk, the twigs, or trunk and outline. Kerschensteiner finds

---

[1] Hanna Rydh, *Grottmänniskornas årtusenden*, p. 130.
[2] Cartailhac et Breuil, "Les peintures et gravures murales des cavernes pyrénéenes". *L'Anthropologie*, 21, pp. 138 *et seq.* Hanna Rydh, *loc. cit.*, p. 130.

the following formalized shapes for trees:[1] 1. The
trunk is drawn and the branches are given as a bundle
of simple undivided, stiff or bent lines (broom formula).
2. The branches are drawn standing out from both sides
of the trunk (feather formula). 3. The outline of the
foliage is shown by a dense or somewhat more open
circular scribble placed at the top of the trunk (coil
formula). 4. The foliage is given as a lobate outline
added to the trunk (lobate formula). All these appear
in Margaret's drawings, and I have observed them in
the drawings of other children. Kerschensteiner also

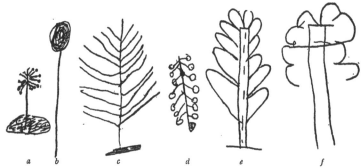

FIG. 119.—TREES. (*a*) BROOM FORMULA; (*b*) COIL FORMULA; (*c*)
FEATHER FORMULA; (*d*) FRUIT TREE IN FEATHER FORMULA;
(*e*) *and* (*f*) LOBATE FORMULÆ. (*a*) FROM KERSCHENSTEINER;
(*b*) *and* (*f*) FROM MARGARET'S DRAWINGS; (*c*), (*d*), *and* (*e*) BY
BEGINNERS AT THE ELEMENTARY SCHOOL IN OSLO.

speaks of a ladder formula—parallel lines drawn across
the trunk, but this cannot be clearly distinguished from
the feather formula (Fig. 119). Later on, the representation is completed by the addition of twigs, leaves, fruit,
etc. The children often draw the roots of the tree,
for they know that they are there, although they cannot
be seen. The oldest and most primitive folk art of
palæolithic times also shows us the tree according to the
feather formula, and having visible roots.[2]

In the case of flowers, Kerschensteiner distinguishes

[1] Kerschensteiner, *loc. cit.*, p. 173, Plates 60, 61.
[2] Hanna Rydh, *loc. cit.*, p. 124.

three formulæ which appear to have general validity :
1. The flower appears at the upper end of the stem as
a dense circular scribble or a circle (button formula).
2. The flower is put together from a circle and a wreath
of leaves arranged around it (compound formula or
daisy formula). 3. The flower is bell-shaped (tulip
formula). The two last-named formulæ often have
stalks decorated with᷈ leaves ; this is less common in
the case of the button formula. Margaret uses all three
forms, and in addition, a leaf formula, but the button
formula and the daisy formula appear to be most liked ;
the tulip formula is rarer. Kerschensteiner also mentions

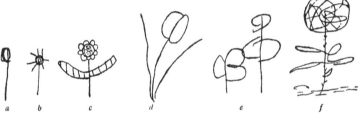

FIG. 120.—FLOWERS. (a) BUTTON FORMULA ; (b) and (c) DAISY
FORMULA ; (d) TULIP FORMULA (BELL FORMULA) ; (e) LEAF
FORMULA ; (f) ROSE FORMULA. (a), (b), (d) and (e) FROM MAR-
GARET'S DRAWINGS ; (c) DRAWN BY BEGINNERS AT THE ELEMEN-
TARY SCHOOL IN OSLO ; (f) FROM KERSCHENSTEINER. 5/6.

a rose formula, which appears not infrequently along
with the other forms (Fig. 120).[1]

The first and favourite subject that children draw is
human beings, but next to that, according to my observations, the house in which they live. They begin with
the façade of the house, which in its most primitive
form is drawn simply as a quadrilateral or rectangle,
with or without windows, without a roof, and often
also without a door. When they reach a higher stage,
they draw windows, door, and roof, this being mostly
shown as a triangle or a trapezium, but sometimes also
as a rectangle or a semi-circle. They rarely forget to
show several ample masses of smoke pouring out from

[1] Kerschensteiner, loc. cit., p. 162, Plates 52, 53.

the chimneys on the roof. Ricci thinks that this preference of children for smoke rising from chimneys, locomotives, tobacco-pipes, etc., depends upon the strong
impression made by the fantastic movement of the
column of smoke upon the little artists.[1] But technique
also plays a part, for the smoke can be represented
with such delightful ease by long spiral or other scribble.

The child's houses are gradually fitted out in greater
and greater detail—it adds staircases, tiles on the roof,
curtains and flowers in the windows. Very often we
are allowed a view of the interior of the house, we see
tables, chairs, and other necessary objects which the
child supposes to exist in every house, and hence must
also be drawn ; furthermore, the inhabitants of the house
appear, they stand up next to their house, or they are
seated inside at table, they stand in a doorway or look
out of a window, or they are also shown floating in
the air in the middle of the house. The house, too, is
beautified by a garden with flowers and trees, a garden
path and often a flag-staff and a fence.

At first children usually draw the house from one
side only, but as they know that the house has several
sides they go on to attempt to show these as well. When
they have acquired some elementary knowledge, they
only draw the two sides that they can really see, often
with some sort of attempt at true perspective representation. But the child very frequently draws three sides.
Ricci asks why these should be three. " Because there
is no possibility and no way of drawing all four."[2]
Both gables are then, as it were, spread out, and drawn
in the same plane as the front side. The shape of the
gabled walls is generally correct, but frequently only
the lower part is drawn as two rectangles, and it also
happens that the lower part is missing and only the
triangular pointed upper part is visible (Fig. 121).

The house is an early and favourite model for the
child, because it is interested in it and has a well-formed

[1] Ricci, *loc. cit.*, p. 35.   [2] Ricci, *loc. cit.*, p. 19.

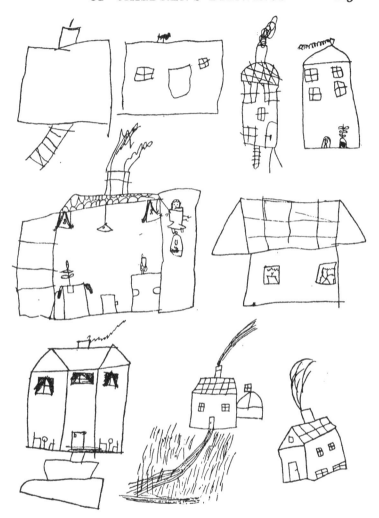

Fig. 121.—The House. Drawn by Beginners at the Elementary School in Oslo. 1/2.

mental picture ; also, it can be represented by simple and divided rectangles, which are so familiar to the child.

F. Rosen points out that the house, which is so closely related to the chief object of representative art, the human figure, plays an important part, not only in children's drawings, but also in primitive art ; this can be seen in the early Renaissance of the thirteenth century, while the representation of houses becomes rarer in the fourteenth century, and in the fifteenth, when art had lost its childlike character, it disappears almost entirely. Like the child, primitive artists represented the house from the front and made its wall transparent so that one could see the life and action of the people inside it. An example of this is seen in Giotto's " The Pope's Dream " in the Monastery Church at Assisi, and in " Zacharias in the Temple " in Santa Croce in Florence.[1] The railway, tram, motor-car and cart, which are all favourite models of children, are allied in form and mode of representation to the house.

All sorts of useful objects, for example, tables, chairs, cups, umbrellas, sledges, etc., gradually appear in the child's repertory. The little draughtsman generally succeeds in producing better representations of them than of models taken from the organic world, no doubt because such useful objects which the child attempts to represent have more simple and regular forms. Its faults are made chiefly in the matter of perspective.

The free drawing of children before the school age is almost entirely from memory, and for the most part it remains the same during the early years at school. Children do not look at the things that they wish to represent, but draw them out of their heads from their mental picture of them. If they are given a model and asked to draw it, the drawing is in most cases very little, or not at all, influenced by the model ; instead, they unhesitatingly follow their memory picture. Kerschensteiner set children of various ages in a Munich school to draw one of their schoolmates in profile turned to the left. 360 out of 1,124 drew the head full face, and 22 with the profile turned to the right.[2] Out of 1,401

---

[1] F. Rosen, *Darstellende Kunst im Kindesalter der Völker*, pp. 18, 19.
[2] Kerschensteiner, *loc. cit.*, p. 34.

formalized drawings, the sitting model was drawn standing in 815. Although children draw mainly in a formalized manner, their products nevertheless do sometimes show features derived from the model, for example, if the latter has a hat on its head or is sitting with folded hands, etc.[1] Kerschensteiner found by comparative experiment that the graphical expression derived from the mental picture was better in most cases than that drawn from nature, and that during the whole school life, drawings from memory were not inferior to drawings from the model.[2]

Why does a child draw from memory? This question has been answered in various ways. In my opinion, the chief reason must lie in the fact that children's drawing is definitely ideomotive both in its origin and in its early developments. The child learns drawing by repeating lines and forms innumerable times until it has practised them so well that it only needs a stimulus for them to run into its fingers, as it were, and be put on to paper almost mechanically. The child represents objects by using the store of forms which it has mastered, and making suitable modifications and arrangements of them—it draws a house, for example, with the aid of rectangles which it has already practised. The required alterations and combinations must not be too difficult or too numerous, and not too far removed from the mechanism of its drawing practice, otherwise the child cannot manage them. If the child draws freely from memory, it can arrange its models and its mode of representation to suit itself, and these naturally lie within the range which it has already practised. If children are compelled to draw from a model, they have first to grasp a form which is perhaps strange, difficult, or complicated for them. Since drawing proceeds little by little, part by part, they are obliged to analyse the whole mental representation which they have made of the

[1] Lena Partridge, *loc. cit.*, p. 175.
[2] Kerschensteiner, *loc. cit.*, p. 232.

object into its single parts and then picture to themselves each part clearly and accurately. They then have to arrange the separate mental pictures in correct succession, in accordance with the necessary and perhaps completely new motions of drawing. It is clear that we are dealing here with a series of unusually difficult problems. Finally, they have to keep in mind the general view of the whole while the drawing is being done, and manage simultaneously the execution of the detail, while this latter affair alone is a problem of such novelty and difficulty that it needs, for itself alone, the child's undivided attention. Its powers are not equal to over-

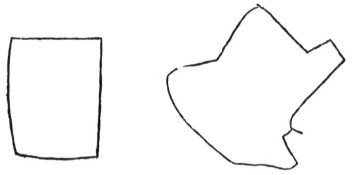

FIG. 122.—RECTANGLE AND RHOMBUS. DRAWN FROM COPIES BY A FIVE-YEAR-OLD GIRL. 1/1.

coming so many new difficulties at one attempt. The child *cannot* draw from nature. It *can* draw from memory, and hence it does do so. That this is a correct statement of the condition is shown by examples from intelligence tests. A test designed for the age of seven years consists in drawing a rhombus from a copy. Here we can observe that younger and less gifted children draw straight and curved lines in all directions; for example, a normally gifted child of five produced instead of the rhombus a tangle of zig-zag strokes, whereas it drew a rectangle with great ease (Fig. 122). A feeble-minded boy of eight could not copy the rhombus but

when he was afterwards given a rectangle, he said with
delight : " Yes, I can draw the house." This was a
form well known to him from scribbling, while the
rhombus is a figure which is new and unaccustomed to
most children who have never drawn it before. It is,
of course, extremely simple in itself, and most normally
gifted seven-year-old children are able to bring about
the necessary co-ordination between concept and movement. These examples teach us that naturalistic drawing apart from unusual artistic gifts demands greater
maturity and talent than formalized drawing from
memory.

How do children draw from memory ? We already
know : they draw in a formalized manner. The next
question must then be : why do children draw in this
way ? This question has also been answered : because
they cannot draw naturalistically. Children cannot
reproduce any model naturalistically, neither the model
which is placed in front of their eyes nor the mental
pictures of the objects which we must assume to be
present in their consciousness. But it would still be
false to say that children draw without models. They
always have them, in part inwardly, in part outwardly.
Their most important subjects are their own earlier
drawings ; they are able to reproduce these naturalistically. These subjects are both internal and external ;
the children see their own drawings, and the motions
which they need to execute them, while in their memory
they have the pictures of their form and of the corresponding motion, and all this forms a structural whole.
Of other external models or objects they are only able
to produce such single features as can be represented by
forms which they have practised in drawing and
scribbling, or such which can be produced by small
alterations and combinations. The same is true of their
inward pictures, their mental representations of objects.
It is just these adaptations and combinations which
bring about progress in drawing and enrich the store of

firmly fixed forms. The child sees how a watch or a ball is drawn, gradually imitates form and movement, and circular scribbling develops from wavy scribbling. It discovers in its scribbling round forms and straight lines, and these can be made use of to represent a human figure. They suffice, it is true, only for some of the most important features, such as the round face and the legs, given by a circle and two straight lines. A few years later, it draws a human figure by making a circle for the face, two circles for the eyes, straight lines for nose and mouth, a circle for the body, and straight lines for arms and legs. The graphic forms are thus the same. What has been the cause of the development which has taken years to come about? Why is the human formula now so much more naturalistic? This must depend mainly upon general mental development : a more complete grasp of impressions, clearer and better defined mental pictures, a better memory, greater power to analyse mental pictures into their constituent parts and yet retain a grasp of the whole, the power to make better co-ordination between mental pictures and movements. The child sees more in its mind that it can draw, just as was the case at an earlier age, for it is still confined to the use of a limited number of formalized shapes which it has practised for expressing itself graphically.

The child draws by making use of its mental pictures of objects. What is the nature of these mental pictures? We might suppose that the child preserves in its memory faithful and accurate pictures of objects so that it only needs to project these, as it were, upon the paper. As Bühler has pointed out, this cannot be the case, for the child could not then bring together in its drawings details which do not in reality appear together,[1] for example, two eyes in a profile or things in the interior of a house seen through the outside wall.

Even if children could retain the mental picture and

[1] *loc. cit.*, pp. 155, 156.

overcome technical difficulties they would not as a rule be able to draw naturalistically. Their mental pictures are, as has been shown by investigation, in no way clear and distinct, but on the contrary blurred and incomplete. Margaret wanted to draw the Norwegian flag correctly and also possessed the necessary technique for doing so, but the mental picture failed and the drawing was formalized. She knew, however, that the flag had some red in it and expressed this knowledge formally by putting a red cross next to the blue cross.

This leads us to another peculiarity of formalized children's drawings, expressed in the rule so often quoted : " Children draw what they know, not what they see."

Even when children have the objects in front of their eyes they generally do not draw what they see but what they know. D. Katz set five- to seven-year-old children to draw from models a four-sided surface with four legs in the form of a table, a cylinder, and so on. All of them drew the table as a rectangle with four lines going outwards or inwards from the corners or four lines going outwards from one of the sides. A three-sided pyramid was produced by three or four sides being put together anyhow. Copies drawn in perspective which were afterwards given to them produced much the same result.[1]

The fact that children draw what they know instead of what they see can be explained, according to Bühler, from a certain general law of our imagination. We have, namely, a tendency to hold fast to certain fundamental forms of objects, their characteristic, or " orthoscopic ", forms. The orthoscopic form of a rectangular table-top is a rectangle, hence children draw the table-top as a rectangle, and it is difficult for them to see it in perspective as a trapezium or a rhombus. Or, to quote Bühler's examples : " Why do the eyes and the mouths of persons appear so frequently full face, while the nose and feet (often in the same figure) are shown in profile ;

---

[1] D. Katz, " Ein Beitrag zur Kenntnis der Kinderzeichnungen ", *Zeitschr. für Psychologie*, 41 (1906), pp. 241 *et seq.*

why are the hands always seen flat ? Because these are obviously the orthoscopic forms of the organs in question." [1]

D. Katz tries to explain how the child comes to prefer the orthoscopic form. A square surface, in order to be seen as square, must be in a position at right angles to the line joining it to the observer, so that the lines of fixation of the eyes are symmetrical. This case therefore differs physiologically from others. It also differs psychologically, since the object is best grasped in this manner. If a rectangular surface, for example a picture, is not in this position, we move it until it is, in order to be able to see it clearly. Hence the rectangular surface is preferred in this form to all the other innumerable forms which it can assume from various points of view. Further, in this form all the others are represented. Here, also, the sense of touch plays an important part. This working out of dominant forms takes place in the earliest years of life.[2]

H. Volkelt shows that we are not always dealing with the orthoscopic form in the drawing of children, but sometimes with a primitive concept of totality, as, for example, when his daughter drew a cube as a circle with four rays sticking out of it—these being the corners of the cube, the circle representing the cube as a whole. Other children drew a cylinder as an oval, for this expressed a straight part and the rounding of the ends and sides, and frequently also the standing or rolling of the cylinder. Volkelt also points out that children draw neither merely what they see, nor only what they know, but also its content of will and feeling.[3]

It is, of course, true that a child's drawing is the expression of its feelings, its strivings, and we might add, the play of its imagination with objects, its æsthetic sense, etc. But the well-known rule is nevertheless

[1] Bühler, *loc. cit.*, pp. 157, 158.
[2] Katz, *loc. cit.*, pp. 249 *et seq.*
[3] H. Volkelt, *Primitive Komplexqualitäten in Kinderzeichnungen*, pp. 204 *et seq.*

correct and explains many of the features peculiar to children's drawings.

It also explains the peculiarity described by Luquet as transparency.[1] Children draw a man on a horse and you see both his legs ; they show someone sitting in a boat and you see the whole figure as if the sides of the boat were transparent. (See Fig. 123.)

This tendency to adhere to the characteristic form of objects appears also in another peculiar feature which may be described as *turning over*, following Luquet, who found many examples of it in Simonne's drawing.[2] For example, the child tries to draw a round pool with trees about it, seen from a point near the shore. It

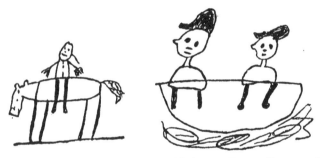

FIG. 123.—A MAN ON HORSEBACK. MEN IN A BOAT. RICCI. 1/1.

gives the trees their physical form, as seen from the side, but nevertheless represented as they would look if they had been cut down and lay with their roots on the shore and tops pointing away from the pool. The pool, also, is not represented true to nature as an oval, but is as it were set upright and drawn in characteristic form as a circle. This last feature might be described, to distinguish it from turning over, as *setting upright*. In a similar way, the top of a table is often set upright and shown as a rectangle, while the table legs are drawn turned over. Simonne drew, even at the age of 7 ; 7, the upper part of a cart set upright, the wheels turned

[1] Luquet, *loc. cit.*, p. 191.   [2] *loc. cit.*, p. 193.

over and completely visible on both sides of the cart. The people sitting in the cart are turned over and lie under the seat, which goes across over their bodies, while the horse appears in characteristic form in side view (Fig. 124). Furniture, the typical appearance of which is best seen in side view, is drawn by Simonne in elevation, including the legs as well. Some girls standing together in a circle she draws turned over, so that they lie in a circle with their feet turned towards one another.[1] Turning over is often seen in children's drawings; thus Bubi, aged 4 ; 7, drew a garden fence turned over.[2] Miss Shinn's niece, aged 5 ; 4, drew a

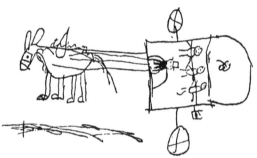

FIG. 124.—DRAWING BY SIMONNE. 7 ; 7. (FROM LUQUET.)

house with turned-over doors, windows, etc.[3] In the case of other children, on the other hand, turning over rarely or never appears, as, for example, Walther-Heinz, Ekki and Günther, of whom nothing of the kind is reported. Margaret's drawings show no trace of it.

This characteristic can be found now and then in the case of adults, who draw rarely or are mentally undeveloped. Two lads, fifteen and sixteen years old, were told to draw the ground plan of a schoolroom, and gave the windows, the doors, the stove, the cupboard, and desks turned over on the floor. This is also to be seen in primitive folk art. In Australian, Egyptian, and Indian

[1] Luquet, *loc. cit.*, pp. 193 *et seq.*   [2] Scupin, *loc. cit.*, II, p. 254.
[3] E. E. Brown, *loc. cit.*, p. 27.

drawings, a pool surrounded by trees is shown set upright, and the trees themselves turned over (Fig. 125). A number of tents standing in a square are shown turned over and so on.[1]

Another characteristic of the child's drawing depends essentially upon the fact that children draw what they know, and not what they see, although in this case an insufficient power of observation and defective technique also play a part. Luquet, in his careful analysis of children's drawing, has described this as a want of synthesis. It appears in side-by-side arrangement, incorrect orienta-

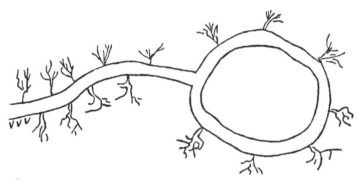

FIG. 125. POOL SURROUNDED BY TREES. AUSTRALIAN BARK DRAWING. (FROM ANDRÉE.) REPRODUCED FROM LEVINSTEIN.

tion, and false synthesis.[2] Side-by-side arrangement denotes that the child draws details which are in reality part of a whole, side by side and distributed over the paper. Simonne, for example, drew a horse and then tried to put its head somewhere else on the paper ; then she drew a house in ground plan, the rooms were put separately on the paper, so that between the outlines of each room and again between these and the outside lines, there was an empty space left. Now and then a room may even be made to lie outside the common outline ;

[1] Levinstein, *loc. cit.*, p. 117 ; Plate 59, Figs. 135–8 ; Plate 60, Fig. 139.
[2] Luquet, *loc. cit.*, pp. 172 *et seq.*

the chimney hangs in the air over a roof, etc. A little
Norwegian girl, Gudrun, four years of age, drew the first
storey of a house as a rectangle, next to it the staircase
to the second-storey bedroom, which was put separately
on the paper ; and finally the " clock-maker " living in

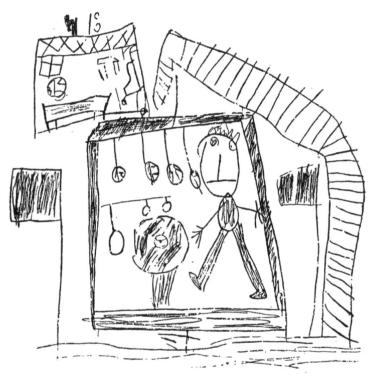

FIG. 126.—THE CLOCK-MAKER. DRAWN BY GUDRUN, 4 YEARS. RED
AND BLUE PENCIL. ABOUT 1/2.

the house, who is of gigantic stature and reaches to the
ceiling of his shop (Fig. 126).

Incorrect orientation appears when the child places its
drawing in a wrong direction with reference to the
surface of the paper or to other parts of the drawing ;
as, for example, when children draw letters wrong side

up or in a horizontal position, or when Simonne draws a man standing on his head in his house.[1]

. Incorrect synthesis is shown when parts of the drawing are arranged together in a manner not in accordance with reality. Simonne sometimes drew the nose below the mouth, another time the nose was put in between hair and eyes ; the door of one of her houses is set on the same side as the chimney in relationship to the windows.[2]

We may also notice that smaller children usually make disconnected and fragmentary pictures, even when they are illustrating a story, while older children often represent its contents in appropriate pictures.

Defective power of synthesis is also a leading characteristic of a child's thinking and talking, indeed of its whole mental life. These same defects appear in palæolithic art even at the period of its highest development ; each model is represented separately, and we rarely see any attempt at even the simplest composition.

Defective synthesis is also characteristic of the drawings of psychically abnormal people. Examples are known of highly gifted artists falling, in a period of mental derangement, to the level of a child's powers, producing pictures consisting of a muddled and disordered mass of details, without any leading idea. Some of the pictures of the Swedish painter Josephson are an example of this.

Bühler points out with truth that the well-known rule, " children draw what they know, not what they see ", while it appears to explain so many peculiar characteristics of children's drawings in a manner both clear and simple, in reality involves the psychological problem, " Is knowing really anything else but mental picturing ? " Bühler answers this question in the affirmative : Judgments are something else besides mental pictures. And judgments, or more exactly speaking, the memory arrangements of judgments, do actually influence the child's drawing.[3]

---

[1] Luquet, loc. cit., p. 178.   [2] Luquet, loc. cit., pp. 180 et seq.
[3] Bühler, loc. cit., p. 157.

We have seen examples of the fact that knowing, that is, an unclear conceptual consciousness of things, properties, and circumstances, influences a child's drawing. Margaret must have *seen* long before she was two and a half years old that a human being has two eyes, but only when the time had come for her to have mastered the numerical concept two, and to *know* how many that is, did she begin to draw persons with two eyes. In such cases it appears as if the mental pictures of the child must crystallize into knowledge in order to acquire such clear outlines that they can be placed on paper. Another example is the formalized expression of Margaret's knowledge that the flag is red. But it would be misleading to describe this knowledge as a judgment, since it is not acquired by the child as a result of logical thinking, but simply by connecting together a number of visual impressions. When the child represents in its drawing of a " flower " the latter's most important characteristics, stem, leaves, petals, this seems like the formalized expression of a logical general concept of wide comprehensiveness.

In actual fact a child's general concept of " a flower " does not come into being through any logical thinking devoted to comparing and distinguishing, but through superficial observation of the most readily noticeable points of similarity between different flowers, leading to an unclearly defined and badly marked concept " flower ". Hence, when Luquet speaks of a " logical realism " of early children's drawing as opposed to the " visual realism " of correct natural representation, this again is misleading. Luquet is quite right in emphasizing the fact that the child strives after realism in its representation, and he supports his views with many examples from Simonne's drawings. But when Luquet explains that earlier writers were labouring under an illusion in characterizing children's drawings as formalized, he is following a false clue.[1] For he entirely failed to take

[1] Luquet, *loc. cit.*, p. 147.

account of the child's scribbling. This scribbling is altogether automatic and is the foundation of those forms which the child develops and applies in representation later on, and it certainly is formalized ; the fact cannot be easily denied. " Formalized naturalism " would be a better expression of the true character of children's drawings than " logical realism ".

F. Rosen speaks of a similar formalized naturalism in primitive art ; thus Giotto gives the leaves of his trees, particularly oak and olive, always in the flat with their characteristic outline, although the upper surface is generally actually turned upwards towards the sky and cannot therefore be seen by the beholder. The same formalized naturalism also appears in the fact that the artist always represents objects fully and completely, even when this representation is far from being true to appearances.[1]

Sully maintains that the child as artist is more a symbolist than a naturalist and that it does not care in the least for complete and exact likeness, but is satisfied with suggestion.[2] If the child only desires a suggestion, it is no doubt because room is left for its imagination to work ; most observers of children's drawing accordingly report that the child derives great pleasure from its own imaginative interpretation of arrangements of lines which it has produced by chance, so long as these have a slight likeness to the mental pictures which they arouse in the child's lively imagination. This symbolism, which actually exists in the child's drawings alongside realism, is paralleled by the symbolism which appears in its play.

Bühler is inclined to see in the child's formalized drawing the result of a process of abstraction, the original conception of the child being concrete and naturalistic, but having become formalized and abstract by the in- fluence of speech and thought. " When the child begins to draw in its third or fourth year, its mental life is

[1] F. Rosen, *loc. cit.*, pp. 19 *et seq.*   [2] Sully, *loc. cit.*, p. 390.

already to a large extent under the dominance of language, and has received from the latter a definite stamp." The child's memory store is at this time no longer a pure collection of mental pictures, but consists in great part of arrangements of judgments which are, or may be, clothed in language. When the child, on commencing to draw, now makes use of its memory store, it does so in a verbalized fashion ; the most important characteristic of this is a certain degree of abstraction, which is necessitated by the very nature of language as a mode of representation.[1] Bühler's view agrees to some extent with Verworn's theory, that the formalization of art depends upon an increasing development of the imaginative life, of abstract theoretical ideas.[2]

The results of the study of the mental development of the child in its first years of life by no means support Bühler's view, that the first childish conception of things is that of a totality true to appearances, though unclear, which later on is formalized in the child's drawings under the compulsion of language. The little girl whose drawing I have carefully followed, began to draw and to speak at about the same time at 1 ; 2 ; at this time she only knew a few words, so that it really cannot be said that her speech had a dominating influence on her drawing. The development of the drawing took place absolutely independently, concomitantly with the development of speech, of the power of forming concepts, of acting, etc. Everything begins automatically, formalized, unordered ; advances, and finally becomes determined by reality, logical, synthetic. The formalized drawing of a child is in accordance with its mental development.

I should also like to mention other influences which might lead the child to draw in a formalized manner. This often happens from indolence, because it wishes to avoid the trouble of making a naturalistic representation. Children leave out lines which they consider purposeless,

---

[1] Bühler, *loc. cit.*, pp. 185 *et seq.*
[2] Verworn, *Zur Psychologie der primitiven Kunst*, p. 727.

as when Margaret spares herself the trouble of drawing arms when her people have nothing for them to do, while she puts arms in when they have to be used. Formalized drawing also often springs from the child's conservatism, in much the same way that children wish to hear a fairy story always told in exactly the same manner. For this reason children's drawing has often been described as conventional formalism (*konventioneller Schematismus*).

AUTOMATISM

After a sufficient number of repetitions, the process of drawing finally becomes quite mechanical. It becomes an automatism. The child when drawing tends to repeat simple automatized movements rhythmically and frequently. Even more complex drawings, whole scenes or landscapes, are produced again and again in the same form:[1] Margaret also gave a few examples of this, though not very many, as her drawings were usually altered on repetition and hence not produced quite automatically.

Rouma observed a number of phenomena connected with automatism. When a movement is automatized, it is made more quickly and easily, but since an impulse of equal strength is often behind it, it is repeated more frequently than is necessary. A somewhat unintelligent boy of seven drew horses and quickly made both pairs of legs in the form of two lines crossing one another; the movement was automatized, and then he began to draw three pairs, and later four. Another unintelligent seven-year-old boy drew his formalized human figures with five carefully-drawn fingers by looking at his own fingers and counting them. Little by little, however, the lines for the fingers were made quickly and automatically, and he gradually increased their number to ten or even twelve on each hand. Another boy produced hands with six or seven fingers and finally indicated

[1] Rouma, *Le langage graphique de l'enfant*, Brussels, 1913, p. 208. Krötzsch, *loc. cit.*, pp. 88 *et seq.*

them by only three quickly drawn lines.[1]   In Margaret's drawings, the "lamp-post" figures and the "cape" figures were perhaps in part the result of her facility in drawing long and straight lines.

As the automatization of the movements of drawing increases, it sometimes happens, as Rouma has shown, that consciousness of their original purpose is weakened. A separation between idea and representation takes place, and this finally leads to degeneration of form and movement. A normally intelligent boy of five and a half drew the facial features of his formalized person and counted them out loud as he did so. The movements gradually became more rapid and their designation rarer, until he finally only drew dots in an ever-increasing number without any order or meaning. They no longer had anything to do with the features of the face.[2]

Automatism also appears when the child, while passing on to a new form, still clings to the old one. According to Rouma, it may also account for the child putting two noses on the face, one in profile, and for it giving a profile two eyes, or representing a bird with four legs.

When a motive is frequently drawn and repeated in the same form, a strong and lasting association is formed between the serial order of the form and the movements of drawing, sometimes hindering the production of new connections. Rouma tells us of a seven-year-old abnormal boy, who had practised the capital Roman P for some time. When he was asked to draw a lady, he produced a P, and he drew this letter in rows when he was asked to copy the name Adrian. A weak-minded boy drew in his book the word POP in big Roman letters. When he came to the letter O, this reminded him of a head, and he automatically drew a body underneath it and put eyes, nose and mouth in.[3]

When simple or even more complex drawings, sometimes whole scenes and landscapes, are often repeated in

---

[1] Rouma, *loc. cit.*, p. 204.   [2] *loc. cit.*, p. 206.
[3] *loc. cit.*, p. 207.

the same form, they may become completely stereotyped pictures, a sort of block (in the printer's sense), as it were. Krötzsch would like to reserve the word " formal " for this stage of children's drawing, but the expression " block " used by Rouma puts more emphasis on the unalterability ; the word " formula " fits the whole of children's drawings, for it expresses their simplified representation of objects.

When the block appears, all development of the child's drawing comes to an end, either temporarily or permanently ; the teacher should therefore do his best to set forces in motion to help the child to cease making blocks and develop further the motives which it has acquired. Very often the child itself does so on its own initiative after having been satisfied for a time with a block-like formula.

Krötzsch proves that not all forms are stereotyped with equal rapidity in the drawing of a child. Things that it sees more rarely, such as birds, fishes, etc., more easily fall a victim to block-like representation than things which the child is always seeing, and busy with. Thus, talented children work as a rule steadily at the improvement of their human figures, and if these finally become stereotyped, they are usually as far advanced as those of moderately gifted adults. The block form appears sooner in the case of less gifted children than in talented ; in the case of children of great talent, it never appears, and their drawings are always alive and capable of development.[1]

Rouma regards automatism mainly as a sign of degeneration, a fact connected with the nature of his investigations ; they were carried out for the most part on unintelligent children. Krötzsch, however, lays more emphasis than others do upon the meaning of automatism and rhythm as fundamental processes in the child's drawing. Form, writing, and ornament develop upon the basis of the first rhythmical and first automatic

[1] Krötzsch, *loc. cit.*, pp. 88 *et seq.*

scribbling of the child. On the other hand, he maintains that form again gives way to motion as interest diminishes and the will weakens ; the form is enlarged and coarsened, sharply marked corners are lazily rounded off, straight lines are drawn crooked, etc.[1] I made the same observation ; a house drawn by Margaret is reproduced here, in which particularly some of the lower windows show degenerated characteristics, while two or three of

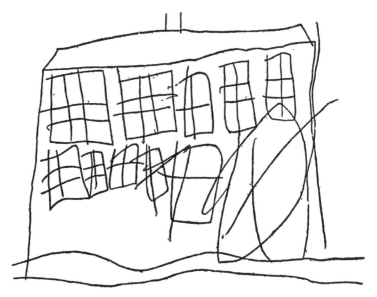

FIG. 127.—AN EXAMPLE, HOW FORM IS LOST WHEN INTEREST DIMINISHES. MARGARET. ABOUT 2/3.

the upper windows are carried out in the usual manner (Fig. 127). Krötzsch states that automatism rules in the drawing of abnormal and mentally deranged persons, and that it also can appear in normal adults when in a state of diminished consciousness ; if one is bored with a lecture, or telephoning, and so on, one begins quite automatically to draw various simple lines and figures,

[1] Krötzsch, *loc. cit.*, pp. 50 *et seq.*

which are repeated rhythmically without any representative intention.[1]

My observations lead me to see great value in automatism for the drawing of the normal and healthy child. *Automatism is not only beginning and degeneration, it is fundamental to every new advance in form and expression ; the repetition and practice which it brings lead to new progress. It is a fundamental process which upholds and supports the whole artistic development of the child.*

ORIENTATION

Want of correct power of orientation is a characteristic in early children's drawing. This weakness in the child's power of representation appears in varied forms. The child brings parts of a single mental picture together in an incorrect relationship to one another. This happens, for example, when the child represents its first human being as a circle standing for both head and body, a number of " eyes " in the middle of the circle, and somewhere in the outline a pair of legs or a few strokes as hairs (incorrect synthesis) ; or when Madeleine, age 5,[2] scatters a roof, four windows and a door, all separated from one another, over the paper, and supposes that she has drawn a house (side-by-side arrangement). Children place objects which belong together as parts of a thing, a landscape, etc., on the paper without any relationship to one another, or even join them together in a way which does not correspond to reality. For example, children illustrate stories by means of fragments of pictures (defective capacity for synthesis). Many such cases of incorrect orientation appear in children's drawing and they may be explained by the rule which we have quoted so frequently : Children draw what they know, not what they see.

Another effect of the failure in the child's sense of orientation is a peculiar phenomenon which, though

---

[1] Krötzsch, *loc. cit.*, pp. 61 *et seq.*, 65 *et seq.*
[2] Rouma, *loc. cit.*, pp. 106, 107.

well known, is very difficult to explain. Every teacher
of a beginners' class must have observed that the children
often write letters and figures upside-down, or in mirror
hand. Less frequently it happens that the letters, as
in Margaret's first attempt, are placed horizontally or at
an angle upon the paper.

We also see this quite frequently in the case of
children's drawing. Stern's daughter, Eva, drew at the
age of three a face, beginning with an oval outline,

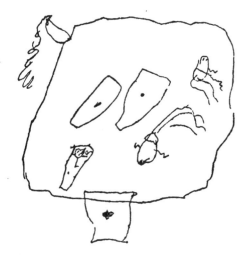

FIG. 128.—HOUSE WITH TWO FIGURES, ONE INVERTED. SIMONNE.
4 ; 2, 24. (FROM LUQUET.)

two eyes at the bottom, then the nose, and the mouth
at the top.[1] Simonne drew human beings by preference
standing on their heads, and trees, horses, dogs, etc.,
likewise upside-down (Fig. 128).[2] Rouma reports that
in the case of several normal and intelligent children,
three to five years old, their human figures were drawn
standing on their heads, horizontal, or at an angle.[3]

[1] W. Stern, " Über verlagerte Raumformen ", *Zeitschrift für angewandte Psychologie*, 2, p. 511.
[2] Luquet, *loc. cit.*, pp. 178, 73.
[3] Rouma, *loc. cit.*, pp. 106 *et seq.*

Albien gave scholars of the age of nine to eighteen years a pattern of lines to draw, partly from memory, partly from copies. Some of them produced a mirror picture, and 18 per cent. of the boys of nine to thirteen years of age drew it horizontal instead of upright, in one case even with the copy alongside; no horizontal drawing was found among the older boys.[1]

Many children learn spontaneously to write a mirror hand with the left, and frequently also with the right hand.[2] Stern had his son age six draw a sailing-ship from memory; and then he gave him the task of drawing it upside-down, and then at an angle of 90°. The result was that he drew both with equal facility. It has been observed that children comprehend pictures almost equally as well when inverted as in a correct position.[3]

The reason for this spatial displacement is not clear. It has been supposed to depend upon disturbances in the innervation of the muscles or upon the inversion of the image on the retina, which children have not yet learnt to understand correctly. The reason is now, however, sought chiefly in our comprehension of space, which according to the latest investigations appears to be partly the result of our experience and connection of images; it is, in other words, learned and not inborn, at any rate not to the extent once assumed.

It is well known that our comprehension of the third dimension of depth and distance away is not completely inborn and quite infallible. We only gradually acquire some certainty in judging the greater or less distance of an object, and we do this by definite signs. It appears smaller at the greater distance, its outlines become less clear, near objects cover up more distant ones, lines approach one another by perspective as the distance increases, etc. Hence we can also make mistakes in regard to distance; when in the mountains, for example,

[1] E. Meumann, *Vorlesungen zur Einführung in die experimentelle Pädagogik*, Second Edition, 3, pp. 732 *et seq.*
[2] Stern, *loc. cit.*, pp. 502 *et seq.*, 512.
[3] *loc. cit.*, pp. 516 *et seq.*

outlines are seen more clearly on account of the mountain air, and we suppose everything to be nearer than it really is.

More recent investigators find that our comprehension of the first two dimensions of surface is similar to our comprehension of depth. As the result of experience, we order our sense impressions on a surface, inasmuch as we place them in space with reference to ourselves. That is above, after which we have to stretch up our arms, that is to the right to reach which we have to stretch our arms to the right ; the things are above, the image of which is projected on to a definite spot of the retina, those are at the right the image of which falls on another spot, etc. Jaensch maintains that there is probably no fundamental difference between comprehension of depth and comprehension of surface. The latter is fixed more quickly than the former, and the difference, so he thinks, depends on a certain inborn disposition, further supported by the fact that the retina is a surface upon which impressions can be ordered.[1]

In this connection the well-known Stratton experiment is interesting. He bandaged one eye and placed before the other a combination of lenses having the effect of inverting the image on the retina. The world appeared to him standing on its head ; at first he found himself in great confusion in all his movements, in dressing, eating, etc., he had to battle with the greatest difficulties ; when he reached for something to the right, it was on the left, what he supposed was above, was below. But in a few days he was already beginning to feel at home in his new surroundings, and in the course of a week he was able to move in an inverted world without any difficulties.[2]

A further result of this is, that our comprehension of single forms in space and on surfaces is not indissolubly

[1] E. R. Jaensch, *Über den Aufbau der Wahrnehmungswelt*, p. 175.
[2] G. M. Stratton, " Vision without Inversion of the Retinal Image ", *Psychological Review*, 4, 1897, pp. 341-60, 463-81.

and infallibly connected with our comprehension of the surrounding space. It is further 'maintained that our comprehension of single space forms is more original and firmer than that of their orientation in space ; this latter is dependent in a high degree upon experience, and hence still uncertain in the case of children. This explains why they turn their letters and drawings in many different directions with reference to the surface of the paper. To take an example, we are accustomed to see a tall and narrow window on the wall of a house always in the same position ; as a space form, however, the window does not necessarily always have this position ; as long as it is in the carpenter's workshop it may be turned into all sorts of directions. But on the wall of the house we are so accustomed to seeing it in this particular position that it never occurs to us to think of it otherwise. In the case of children, this association between window and wall is not yet so firmly ingrained, and this is expressed in their drawing. Günther drew at 4 ; 6, a house with a door and six windows. The house itself, the door and two windows were in the correct position, but four windows, although correct in form and spacing, were drawn in a horizontal position.[1]

In the same way, for example, the position of letters on paper is in our case a firmly fixed association, but not in the case of the child. Even in the case of adults this association is not indissoluble. Type-setters, who have the type before them in a reversed position while working, learn very quickly to read it also in this position. Further, the interest of the child is initially directed particularly towards the form of the letters, since it is trying to impress this upon itself. The tendency exists in ourselves to hold firmly to the single space form.[2] The impulse of attention also plays a part. When a child, for example, has begun at first to draw a letter wrongly, the further course of its attention receives a definite direction from this first impulse, and the form

[1] Stern, *loc. cit.*, pp. 506, 507.   [2] Jaensch, *loc. cit.*, p. 176.

now appears correctly, but the orientation on the surface is sacrificed. Hence it is that spatial displacement in children's drawing and writing always appears with the beginner, and disappears with progressive practice of the association. In the case of children who are naturally of marked visual type, spatial displacement is believed to occur more frequently, since they have more intense experience of spatial form as such.[1] Thus Jaensch was able to produce spatial displacement experimentally in the case of his " Eidetics ".[2] An observation of Jaensch's is interesting in this connection. In the case of one of his experimental subjects he found spatial displacement to occur in the case of objects which are able to change their position in actual fact, as, for example, human beings, but not in the case of objects such as rocks and trees, which are by nature immovable. Spatial displacement in the case of these, if it nevertheless occurred by way of exception, was generally in the form of the mirror image.[3]

Other causes may also contribute to the production of spatial displacement in the drawing and writing of children. For example, incorrect orientation may frequently occur on account of the available space on the paper. Stern reports the case of a five-year-old boy, who was able to write both mirror and ordinary script with either hand, though mirror-writing, which he learned first, was easiest for him ; he wrote mirror-writing when he began to write on the right-hand side of the paper. Once he wrote a letter quite correctly from left to right, but when he came to the signature, and presumably had a dim notion that this was always placed at the right, he commenced writing on the right-hand side of the paper and wrote the signature in mirror hand.[4] Simonne frequently wrote normally until she reached the right edge of the paper, where she turned round and wrote towards the left in mirror hand. Once, at the age of

---

[1] Stern, *loc. cit.*, p. 525.   [2] Jaensch, *loc. cit.*, pp. 162 *et seq.*
[3] *loc. cit.*, p. 171.   [4] Stern, *loc. cit.*, p. 503.

6 ; 8, she wrote at the bottom of a narrow strip of paper her name, then began at the right and wrote in mirror hand to the left " nomiS " ; when she found no room for the last two letters, she wrote above it in a normal hand towards the right " ne ".[1] Rouma observed that some children drew human figures at one time with the legs upwards, at another with the legs downwards. He found by experiment that when they began at the lower edge of the paper they drew first a circle, the head, and then the legs pointing upwards; when he had them

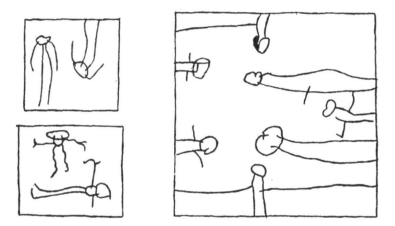

Fig. 129.—Examples of Indifferent Orientation conditioned by the Space Available. Belgian Children, Three-and-a-half Years. (From Rouma.)

begin at the upper edge, the legs were pointed downwards. Others always put the legs on at the point where they had closed the circle, so that they pointed in every possible direction. In the case of eight children, three to five years of age, he observed that they usually drew the legs at the side, where there was most room, while a small child of three and a half years always put the legs on that side where the edge of the paper was nearest to the head (Fig. 129). Rouma sometimes said to the

[1] Luquet, *loc. cit.*, p. 179.

children who drew upside-down : " That man of yours is walking on his head with his legs in the air." Most of the children looked at him with astonishment or laughed at him ; some also pointed to the legs and said : " You see that he has got legs and is walking with them." Rouma points out that a sheet of paper lying on the table has neither a top nor a bottom so that it is quite comprehensible that the children put the legs on their figures in every possible direction. Rouma repeated the experiment with a blackboard and found that the legs in this case were drawn downwards more frequently than usual, but even in this case they were frequently drawn in all sorts of directions.[1] Stern reports that his children also drew with spatial displacement on a vertical blackboard, and concludes that ignorance of the usual orientation on a sheet of paper is not the only reason for spatial displacement.[2]

Rouma distinguishes between indifferent orientation in which the drawings are made in the most various directions, and reversed orientations where the drawings are always upside-down. He reports two typical cases of the latter description. Two boys, three years old, both normal and healthy children, always drew things upside-down, even on a blackboard. Although they had been educated in a Froebel school and had had their mistakes pointed out to them, they retained this peculiarity for several months.[3]

Alice Dégallier, who taught Negro children in a Mission school, observed in the case of her school children, when they began to write, a strong tendency to write letters and figures inverted or in mirror hand.[4]

Mirror and reversed writing are frequently to be observed according to Rouma in the case of abnormal children.[5] It has been supposed that mirror-writing

[1] Rouma, *loc. cit.*, pp. 106 *et seq.*   [2] Stern, *loc. cit.*, p. 519.
[3] Rouma, *loc. cit.*, pp. 110 *et seq.*
[4] A. Dégallier, " Notes psychologiques sur les Nègres Pahouins ", *Archives de Psychologie*, 4, pp. 362 *et seq.*, 1905.
[5] Rouma, *loc. cit.*, p. 111.

was connected with low mental capacity, but this appears not to be the case, unless perhaps in the case of older children who are unable to observe their mistake and hence find it difficult to correct it. Stern also maintains that it has nothing to do with left-handedness.[1] It is quite normal for adults and children who have practised writing to be able to write mirror hand with the left hand without any practice, on account of the symmetrical motor practice.

Spatial displacement appears generally to occur in the case of younger children ; in the case of older children particularly when they have to execute unaccustomed or difficult forms, such as figures and cursive writing, or a difficult and abstract line pattern such as the one used by Albien.

Rouma discusses the question whether spatial displacement is a psychical anomaly, or whether it may not be simply a normal phenomenon, the visual mechanism not being able, for want of sufficient practice, to place the visual image upright.[2] Since numerous observations have proved that spatial displacement is found in the case of normal and well-endowed children at a certain stage of development, it must be considered as a normal phenomenon within certain limits. It is probable that the reversal of the visual image on the retina has something to do with it, since when displacement takes place, the forms are usually inverted. But this cannot be the only cause, since it does not explain horizontal or oblique displacement. The chief cause of spatial displacement must probably be sought in the fact that the associations between individual spatial forms and surrounding space, or as it might perhaps be expressed, the structural formation of the perceptual world of the child, are less firmly practised in the case of children than in the case of adults. Hence spatial displacement generally occurs in the case of new forms unknown to the child.

[1] Stern, *loc. cit.*, pp. 513, 526.
[2] Rouma, *loc. cit.*, p. 112.

PERSPECTIVE

Children's drawing, like primitive folk art, is the representation of outlines and surfaces, and this is the point at which there is the greatest and least questioned agreement between the art of the child and that of the races of man. Palæolithic art, that of the Bushmen and Eskimos, ancient Egyptian art and Greek vase painting are full of life and motion as compared with the stiff and formalized drawing of children, but they all have one characteristic in common, namely, an incapacity for perspective representation, which was also observable in the Middle Ages and to some extent even in the art of the early Renaissance.

It is quite clear that the first products of the child cannot be correct in perspective when we consider their origin. This lies in wavy scribbling, in the production of pure lines without surface. Then there comes scribbling of circles, rectangles, ovals, zig-zag lines, spirals, and later on, the child produces its formalized and fixed mental images of objects as formalized and fixed surfaces and lines.

Perspective representation requires a capacity for abstraction and complex naturalistic synthesis which is not to be found in younger children. In order to draw a square table in correct perspective, the child must be able to abstract from its formalized mental image of the table-top as a rectangle with equal sides, and it must be able to observe and picture to itself, either intuitively or consciously, that it sometimes looks like a trapezium or a rhombus. In order to be able to draw a house in correct perspective, it must abstract from the two sides which are not visible and from its conception of the side of a house as a rectangle, and must be able to follow the perspective course of the lines, and so on. Experimental investigations have shown that, in the matter of abstraction and manifold synthesis, children are generally but little developed up to the age of fourteen years.[1]

[1] Cf. Helga Eng, *Abstrakte Begriffe im Sprechen und Denken des Kindes.*

Investigations on the comprehension and representation of perspective by children have been carried out by Passy, Clark, Kerschensteiner, Rouma, and others.

Passy made children draw objects which presented difficulties in perspective representation. He found that children do not perceive how the dimensions of objects vary with the distance, and that they do not grasp perspective changes in the form of objects. For example, they draw a book, seen from the front, quite correctly with correct angles and parallel sides. When the book is laid down so that the angles are no longer right angles and one side appears foreshortened, the book is not drawn as accurately as before. It is extremely difficult to get the child to perceive its error. It is of course possible to bring it to see the altered position of the book, but the altered form is incomprehensible to it ; it appears to the child nonsensical that a rectangular object should cease to be rectangular, that the shorter sides should appear the longer, and so on.

Passy found that children often misunderstand pictures of known objects when in strong perspective. A funnel much foreshortened with the point towards the beholder was taken for a bunch of flowers, a flat-iron for a bell, and so on. On the other hand they were able easily to understand representations of objects drawn by other children although incorrect in perspective and almost without any shape. Passy concludes from this that children really believe that they see objects as they represent them.[1]

Clark gave six- to sixteen-year-old children in four different schools a hat-pin to draw, which was stuck through an apple placed in front of the children. A hundred and thirty-seven children drew it visible in its whole length through the apple ; one hundred and fifty only drew the parts visible outside the outline of the apple ; a hundred and twenty-one drew it correctly,

[1] Passy, " Notes sur les dessins d'enfants ", Revue Philosophique, 22, pp. 617 et seq., 1891.

that is to say, with one part passing within the outline of the apple, and the other appearing behind it (Fig. 130).

The sides of the outlines of a book laid sloping on the table were given incorrectly as to number by one hundred and twenty-eight children, sixty-six drew them correct in number but incorrect in their relations, seventy-eight drew only the visible sides in correct relationship to one another. Before the age of seven, children in general make no attempt to draw a book in its correct position with the correct number of sides in true relationship to one another. They draw a formula which corresponds with their mental image of a book ; actuated by a kind of sense of order, they draw it parallel with the edges of the paper. Towards the eighth year feeble signs of

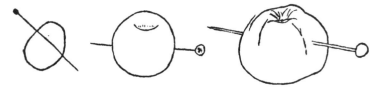

FIG. 130.—THE STAGES OF DEVELOPMENT OF PERSPECTIVE REPRE-
SENTATION. SIX TO SIXTEEN YEARS. (FROM CLARK.)

correct drawing show themselves. At the age of nine, 45 per cent drew the book in its real position, 35 per cent the correct number of sides, and 10 per cent drew the corners fairly correctly. As the age increases progress is seen, and at the age of about fourteen, most were able to give a fairly correct representation of the sides, and half of the children showed the relationship between the sides correctly.[1]

Kerschensteiner summarizes his results with regard to the development of perspective drawing in the following paragraphs :

" The development of the power of expression as regards the representation of a spatial whole does not

[1] Clark, " The Child's Attitude towards Perspective Problems ", *Studies in Education* (Barnes), I, pp. 283 *et seq.*

take place in parallel with that for the representation of a single, self-contained object.

" The first stage of the graphic representation of space is either complete absence of space or the setting of the various objects contained in the space alongside one another."

" The second stage in graphical representation of space includes drawings which are either a conscious attempt at spatial representation, which for one reason or another is not successful, or make the impression of being such an attempt. Here we find map-like representations showing objects turned over in the plane of the paper. We find unsuccessful attempts at bird's-eye view, representations from two or several points of view, simple placing of figures one over the other with continual reduction in size, marking out of space by simple outlines, and so on. Attempts of this kind clearly intended to represent space, but unsuccessful, are found now and then in children as young as six years.

" The third stage is that of successful but incomplete spatial representation. The child makes use of a strip of ground of greater or less width, and expresses his ideas of space by taking perspective foreshortening into consideration and making sparing use of the masking of one object by another. But in all these representations a definite horizon, actually represented or even suggested, is wanting.

" The fourth and last stage is that of the faultless pictorial representation of the whole space. It makes use of all means of line and atmospheric perspective, masking, surface contours, the change in proportions with distance, and the use of shadows and reflected lights." This is very rarely reached before fifteen years of age and then only as the result of imitation.[1]

Rouma draws the following conclusions from his experiment on perspective drawing of children :

[1] Kerschensteiner, " Die Entwicklung der zeichnerischen Begabung ", *Deutsche Kunsterziehung*, pp. 21, 22.

At first the child draws what it knows of a thing, without thinking of what is partially or completely invisible for perspective reasons.

It draws the four wheels of a carriage, one behind the other, or attached to the four corners of the body, represented by a rectangle. It draws all the sides of a house side by side, and human beings are placed in rows.

The second stage is characterized by the placing of several planes one over the other. More distant persons or objects are set out in a plane above the first one. Each plane forms in itself a closed whole. When connections are made between the different planes, the third stage begins.

At the fourth stage, the child finally grasps intuitively the laws of perspective, and takes pains to make use of them, although it still continues to make many mistakes.[1]

At the age of 4 ; 3, 21, Margaret made her first attempt at spatial representation in her drawing " a little girl swinging ", for here four straight lines mark off a portion of ground upon which grass is drawn.

Walther-Heinz drew a ground line at the age of 3 ; 3,[2] Bubi at 5 ; 6,[3] Günther appears to have accomplished it at about 5 ; 0,[4] Ekki at 4 ; 5,[5] Simonne at 4 ; 7, 27.[6]

At 5 ; 11, Margaret began to draw several planes one over another and also to bring them into connection one with another (Rouma's second and third stage). In her drawing " a house in the country " there is a waterfall in the foreground and a path planted with flowers leading at a slope up to the house, and a man walking on it. The house is standing on a broad strip marked off with shading and has trees and flowers on both sides. At 5 ; 11, 7, she produced her drawing of a town house in three planes—at the bottom grass and flowers ; the house stands above this without any connection with it on a ground line planted with flowers

[1] Rouma, *loc. cit.*, p. 129.   [2] Dix, *loc. cit.*, p. 79.
[3] Scupin, *loc. cit.*, 2, p. 258.
[4] Stern, *Die zeichnerische Entwicklung eines Knaben*, p. 13.
[5] Krötzsch, *loc. cit.*, p. 37.   [6] Luquet, *loc. cit.*, p. 110.

and trees ; in the air birds are flying. Thereafter she always made use of several planes in her drawing, and the connecting links between them are always more and more successful. The extent of her final progress is best shown by her drawing of St. Hanshaugen, at the end of the eighth year.

Günther drew a sea picture at the age of 5 ; the surface of the water is shown by a wavy line, below is a diver with helmet and air-pipe, above a steamship, cliffs and fishermen.[1] Walther-Heinz made, at the age of 5 ; 4 and 5 ; 5, two pictures on which a tree, a house, and over them the sky with clouds and stars are to be seen.[2]

It is more difficult to determine from Simonne's drawings the point at which her first combination of several planes appeared, for several of her drawings, which apparently represented several planes, actually are drawn as ground plans with the objects turned over. The real working out of several planes appears to have commenced in her case at the age of 6.[3] Scupin and Krötzsch give no examples in this matter.

A similar placing in " stories " without connection with one another is also seen in primitive folk art, for example, the ancient Egyptian.

Margaret noticed that objects diminish in size with increasing distance at the age of 4 ; 4. One day in the summer holidays, she saw some grown-up people playing croquet at some distance away, and said : " I don't know why they are so small." " When do they become so small ? " " When we are far away from them." At 4 ; 7, she saw the picture of an ant and asked : " Why is it so big ? " It was about twice natural size. Once later on, when she had forgotten what it represented, she called it a wasp. Some days afterwards she saw the picture again, and when I asked her what it was, she said : " That is the ant." " What did you call it before ? " After repeated questions and some considera-

---

[1] Stern, *loc. cit.*, p. 13.   [2] Dix, *loc. cit.*, pp. 87, 90.
[3] Luquet, *loc. cit.*, Plates LXXVI *et seq.*

tion, " I said a wasp," and she laughed at her own stupidity. " Why did you call it that ? " " Of course, because it's so large." At 4 ; 7, 14, she saw the picture of a little boy in the newspaper, and said : " What is that ? " " You see that it is a little boy." " Why is he so small ? " " Do you think he should be larger ? " " Yes, as large as this," and she spread out both arms at full length. When, for example, she saw small pictures of bears or lions, of which she was accustomed to see large ones, she often asked : " Why is it so small ? " In spite of the above-mentioned observations she thus still expected to some extent to see objects pictured in natural size or at least always in the same size. At about 6 ; 2, on several of her pictures, she drew smaller in size what was intended to be farther away.

Stern reports concerning Günther at the age of 5 ; 3½, the following remark, given word for word : " How does it happen that some painters can paint so that it looks as if it was far away ? " When he learnt the reason, he immediately began to make use of his new knowledge, by drawing, in his sea pictures, ships near at hand large, and more distant ones smaller and higher.[1] Vilh. Rasmussen relates of his little daughter : " at the age of 6 ; 1, R. understood the perspective effect of distance. She looked at a picture with a pack of wolves, the last of which were far away. I asked her : ' Why is the last wolf so small ? ' She answered : ' Because it is so far away. It is just as big as the first when it comes quite near.' But in spite of this knowledge her drawings, as has been already related, show hardly any indications of perspective." [2]

The accounts of Bubi and Walther-Heinz (up to the sixth year), of Simonne, Ekki (up to the ninth year), contained nothing which allows us to draw any conclusions in the matter of this characteristic of perspective comprehension.

[1] Stern, *loc. cit.*, p. 14.
[2] Vilh. Rasmussen, *Börnehavebarnet*, pp. 92, 93.

At 4 ; 8, 22, Margaret showed that she knew that the near covers the further ; for she drew only the upper part of the body of a woman who was seen through a window, and explained : " We don't see the other part, for that's down below." We still find, nevertheless, in her later drawings, occasional examples of transparency, although they only occur rarely ; as a rule she shows, quite correctly, that which is in front as hiding that which is more distant. Simonne remarked, as she drew a house at the age of 4 ; 7, 30 : " We don't see the dining-room, that's behind." At 5 ; 2, and 5 ; 9, she only drew the heads of people looking out of the window.[1] Nevertheless, she is guilty of transparency in many other drawings. Günther, at the age of 4 ; 8½, drew a man seen from behind ; when he was told, " Oh, the poor man has no mouth or nose ! " he half turned his back and said : " Do you see the mouth when he's walking like this ? " " But you still see the eye." When on the next day he had drawn a house, he refused to draw a bed in it, saying : " You don't see that in the window, it stands against the wall."[2] Walther-Heinz, at the age of 5 ; 5, drew only the upper part of people looking out of the windows on the railway.[3] At 5 ; 6, Bubi only drew the upper part of the body and one arm of his mother standing at a window and waving, and only the head and fingers of the child lying in its bath and holding on to the edge with its fingers.[4] Krötzsch gives no examples in this connection in his biography.

Margaret first tried to draw single objects in perspective in her street scene, at the age of 6 ; 0, 3, where the two perambulators show an attempt at perspective drawing, as regards the hood, the handle, etc. Masking is also made use of in the representation of the two girls walking behind the perambulator. Here also we found an example of the fact, that children " draw the perspective they know " ; the push-cart shows only two wheels,

[1] Luquet, *loc. cit.*, pp. 210 *et seq.*   [2] Stern, *loc. cit.*, pp. 11, 12.
[3] Dix, *loc. cit.*, p. 89.   [4] Scupin, *loc. cit.*, pp. 258, 259.

which are to be seen clearly on one side, although the two others should also be partly visible. When children draw a dog or a horse with only two legs, this is not always due to their incapacity ; Margaret, aged 6 ; 4, 2, drew a dog, and when I pointed out to her that it only had two legs, she said : " We don't see the other two."

Günther drew houses with two sides from the age of 5 ; 6½ onwards, and at 5 ; 7 he attempted a perspective representation of a reel of cotton, a chair, a table, and a water-bottle, and at 5 ; 8½, a bath-tub. W. Stern points out that this hardly arose from observation, but from unconscious reminiscences of other pictures.[1] Walther-Heinz, at the age of 5 ; 5, made only a few slight attempts to show a locomotive and a house in perspective.[2] From the age of 6 ; 7, Simonne tried to draw houses in perspective ; at 7 ; 1, a pot, and 7 ; 2, a chair,[3] while in most of her other drawings she still made no use of perspective. Bubi made a quite unique attempt at the perspective representation of a staircase.[4] Krötzsch makes no mention of drawings of this kind.

Another characteristic of perspective representation, namely, the approach of lines with increase of distance, I have found only in Margaret's drawings. At 6 ; 2, 3, in her picture of tobogganing, she causes the lines to approach one another as they recede to the background, where there is a house which is shown very small because it is far away. In the drawing of a train at the age of 6 ; 2, 20, also, the rails approach one another in the same manner, and the same little house with small details is to be seen in the background. She began drawing interiors at about 6 ; 8. At first she placed tables, chairs, persons, etc., on a straight ground line. A few attempts at perspective drawing can be seen, for example, a round table, the top of which is shown oval. At 6 ; 9, 10, she drew a room in perspective, with the ceiling

[1] Stern, loc. cit., pp. 19, 21, 24.   [2] Dix, loc. cit., pp. 88, 90.
[3] Luquet, loc. cit., p. 212, Plates CXVI, CXVII.
[4] Scupin, loc. cit., p. 255.

and two side walls foreshortened ; this she called " drawing corners ". When asked where she had learnt this, she answered that she had seen it in her picture-book and that the teacher had also spoken about it ; hence the effect had been produced by copies, which nevertheless would hardly have had any result if she had not been prepared by her earliest attempts at perspective representation. In this room she drew a round table, a rocking-chair, and an ordinary chair, all approximately correct in perspective, while a chest-of-drawers was seen in front view ; all furniture is placed on the front ground line. The lamp on the ceiling was first attached to the front line at the top, then she detected her mistake, rubbed it out and placed it correctly in the middle of the ceiling. At 6 ; 9, 17, she drew a similar interior. A rectangular table and a chair are given in fairly correct perspective. The back legs are even shown shorter than the front ones, but all this is represented from a different point of view than the room itself. When I asked her why she drew the room in this way, she stood against one wall, pointed with both hands at the opposite corners of the ceiling, and said : " When I stand here and look at it like this, it is so, a square, that's surely not a room." Her perspective was therefore fully conscious, and not merely intuitive, or mechanically imitative.

In her eighth year she drew round tables and other round surfaces correctly as ovals, and also drew rectangular surfaces in perspective, but always—without reference to the point of view—as rhombi ; but finally she began to draw a door opening inwards quite correctly as a trapezium. Rectangles, for example a bed, were drawn narrower when foreshortened, without, however, the end lines being made to approach one another.

As far as I can see, she was further advanced for her age in the matter of perspective comprehension and representation than any of the other children whose biography is known to me.

PROPORTIONS

In children's drawings a striking want of correct proportions is noticeable, not only as regards the relationship of the separate parts of an object or a shape to one another, but also in the respective relations of persons and objects in compositions.

The commonest mistake in the child's representation of the human figure is that of making the head too large ; this is also confirmed by the investigations of Schuyten and Lobsien, concerning proportion in children's figure-drawing. Bühler thinks that this can be explained by the human face being especially interesting to the child, all the more because the latter so often has the opportunity of seeing it very close.[1] Lobsien reminds us that the proportions of a child's body are different from those of an adult's, and that the head of a child appears comparatively large.[2] The child pays very little attention to the body of its figures. At first it is omitted altogether, later on it is generally too small, or more rarely, as in the case of Margaret's lamp-post figures, excessively long and thin, or as in her cape-figures, disproportionately broad. The arms are often too long, especially when they are put in for the purpose of showing action of some sort, and need to reach as far as the given position ; but in many drawings they are too short ; the same is true of the fingers. In most children's drawings the legs are too short, in rare cases too long ; the feet are generally too small, but frequently also too long, especially while still shown only by a straight line, as in some of Simonne's drawings. The eyes are at first often so large that they fill the whole circle of the face, and the line of the mouth not infrequently runs right across the face ; the nose is very carelessly treated by children, at least as long as they are drawing full face. It is often entirely left out, or only indicated by a dot

---

[1] Bühler, *loc. cit.*, p. 164.
[2] Lobsien, " Kinderzeichnungen und Kunstkanon ", *Ztschr. f. päd. Psychol.*, 7, 1905, p. 402.

or small circle. When indicated by a line, a triangle, or the like, it is easily made too large. The ears stand out like two large handles on either side of the head. Correct proportions are seen more frequently as a rule in the representation of other objects, than in figures. Children have as a rule a good eye for symmetry, perhaps because it is practised in daily experience in earliest childhood. The child's defective sense of correct proportion is particularly revealed in its compositions of landscapes, situations, etc. People are shown as high as a two-storied house or a church tower, a horse is only half as large as a man, and so on.

The most important reason for this peculiarity in children's drawings is no doubt to be found in their feeble capacity for synthesis ; they cannot, when occupied with drawing the details, retain a grasp of the whole. The parts are drawn piece by piece without taking the total effect into account. Other causes are, however, effective. A child emphasizes in its drawings what appears interesting and important to it, frequently by making it particularly large.[1] Margaret had seen a fairy play and on the next day set to work to draw " Cinderella ". " She was big," she said, and drew a face which covered the whole sheet of paper ; when she noticed that there was no room on the paper for the body, she turned the paper round and drew Cinderella somewhat smaller, but again remarked, " She was big." Rouma gives a number of similar examples.[2] What is new is interesting, hence the child shows features which are new to it disproportionately large in size. Rouma tells us of a boy, six years of age, who put boots on his figures for the first time, whereupon these were drawn with unusually large feet.[3] Bubi, at 4 ; 9, drew his mother for the first time with hands—and made them gigantic.[4] Want of proportion also frequently arises

---

[1] Rouma, *loc. cit.*, pp. 142 *et seq.* ; Scupin, *loc. cit.*, 2, pp. 146, 190.
[2] Rouma, *loc. cit.*, p. 142.   [3] *loc. cit.*, p. 76.
[4] Scupin, *loc. cit.*, 2, p. 146.

from want of room.[1] Margaret, at 6 ; 9, 10, drew a lady
with a large head and much too small body right at the
bottom of the paper ; when I pointed this out to her,
she said : " I hadn't any more room." It also happens
that children are led to draw consciously and intentionally out of proportion through being carried away, as it
were, by artistic delight at a characteristic line or by a
sense of the humour of comic exaggeration. As examples
of the first case we may take Margaret's " lamp-post
figures " and " cape figures " ; and also her stylized
three-cornered houses. Examples of the second motive
may be found in the writings of Rouma, Krötzsch, and
other authors.[2]

Ricci has already pointed out that the want of a sense
of proportion is a common characteristic of children's
art, primitive art, and degenerate art.[3] Figures with
heads too large and bodies too small and figures that are
taller than the towers and keeps of castles alongside
them, are also seen on pictures from the Middle Ages.

Rosen shows that errors such as are most frequently
seen in children's drawings still appear in the art of the
early Renaissance—human figures represented too large
relatively to their surroundings, houses, trees, mountains.
On Giotto's picture, " The Pope's Dream ", St. Francis
is almost as tall as the tower of the Lateran Basilica,
and he would not be able to pass through the church
door, as his height is half as great again as the door.[4]

The same causes are at work here as in children's
drawing, namely, a want of general view and synthetic
power. In primitive folk-art, likewise, that which is
interesting and meaningful is particularly emphasized.
Rouma gives us some example of this. In a Bushman's
drawing of a fight between Bushmen and Kaffirs, the
latter are represented as of gigantic stature compared
with the Bushmen, probably as an expression of the

[1] Luquet, *loc. cit.*, p. 62.
[2] Rouma, *loc. cit.*, pp. 177 *et seq.* ; Krötzsch, *loc. cit.*, p. 82.
[3] Ricci, *loc. cit.*, p. 29.   [4] Rosen, *loc. cit.*, pp. 9 *et seq.*

importance ascribed to the hereditary enemies of the race. Another Bushman's drawing shows a man fighting with a wild animal of greatly exaggerated size. Rouma also mentions a picture by Fra Angelico, in which St. Peter addressing the people is represented ; the Apostles Peter and Paul are giants among a race of pigmies.[1]

MOVEMENT

One of the weakest points in children's drawing is the representation of movement and action. The first formulæ for human beings and animals are stiff and expressionless, with rigid bodies and stiff, immovable limbs. The child's attempts to express posture and gesture appear gradually, but development in this respect is slow and difficult, and only the more gifted children get so far as to be able to show gestures and actions more or less satisfactorily.

Rouma investigated the child's power of representing motion in the case of a number of children, whose exercises in drawing he followed very carefully for at least a couple of years. He distinguishes four stages in the child's representation of motion.

At the first stage the child shows all persons in a neutral position. They are all alike and have the same stereotyped expression. The child nevertheless often imagines that they are performing certain actions, and describes these with words and gestures.

At the second stage, the child represents a partial motion in the form of a connection. For example, he lengthens the arm of a person by a line drawn to another person or thing, which are the objects of the action. The arm thereby becomes disproportionately long, particularly when the connecting line, as frequently happens, is added after the drawing is finished. Thus, a little girl represents a boy plucking apples by drawing a line from the hand of the boy to the tree.

At the third stage, the child attempts to represent

[1] Rouma, *loc. cit.*, p. 78, footnote ; p. 248.

independent partial movements of single persons or animals, that is to say, not as in the second stage between two persons, etc. Children attempt to reproduce movements as they have actually seen them, for example, those of a man walking or clapping his hands, or looking up to the sky, etc.

At the fourth stage, the child endeavours to give a complete representation of posture, motion and actions in their totality. When children have finally opened their eyes to motion, they continually observe it in their surroundings and take great care to reproduce it correctly, so that they are frequently successful in representing motions and actions correctly and characteristically.[1]

Margaret's first attempt to represent an action is her drawing of the little girl swinging at the age of 4 ; 3, 21. We see the little girl on the swing, it is true, but arms and legs stick out beyond it stiffly and rigidly. The motion is only expressed in words. At 4 ; 6, she drew a boat and then said : " The *fjord* is going over it," whereupon she represented the wave motion by circular scribble. The next attempt is her drawing of God carrying a soul up to Heaven, in which God's extended arm indicates the action of carrying up (at 4 ; 8, 22). The drawing of a little girl climbing up a staircase into Heaven, which was done about the same time, is quite formalized and shows no attempt at representing motion. On the other hand, in the drawing " a country house " at 5 ; 11, a man walking towards the house is shown.

In the picture " all the dolls are tobogganing ", at 5 ; 11, 13, she indicates, it is true, that the dolls are holding the toboggan rope but the hands are still formalized and drawn with outspread fingers. In her street picture at 6 ; o, 3, progress in the representation of motion is to be seen. Two ladies, each pushing a perambulator, are grasping with their hands the handles of their perambulators, and a little girl is walking alongside one of the perambulators and holding on to it with one

[1] Rouma, *loc. cit.*, pp. 86 *et seq.*

hand. A hand holding something is now represented for about a year as a small dense circular scribble. At 6 ; 1, 20, Margaret drew a sitting figure for the first time —" Mother with Margaret on her lap ". Mother has her arms round Margaret and folds her hands in a circular scribble. At 6 ; 2, 3, Father, Mother and Margaret are sitting on a sleigh.

A drawing of seated figures is very difficult for children. None of the other five children, whose drawings were observed up to the age of six years or longer, ever represented persons seated. Simonne still showed them stretched out straight in carriage or boat at the age of nine. Lena Partridge, who had some hundred school children of various ages draw a sitting model, reports that the younger children drew a figure standing upright, as though they had simply not seen the one sitting down.[1] Of 1,401 formalized drawings of a seated figure, Kerschensteiner found 815 which had not taken notice of the sitting position.[2] F. Rosen points out that even Italian painters in the fourteenth and fifteenth centuries still frequently had difficulties with the correct representations of sitting or recumbent figures. " In the middle of the fifteenth century Antonio del Pollajuolo tried in vain to draw a seated figure, ' Prudence ', in the Uffizi Gallery in Florence. The legs bent at the knees are fairly correct, but the body is standing, and not sitting." [3]

At 6 ; 3, 1, Margaret, in her picture of the girl swinging and two little girls standing beside her waiting, represented posture and motion fairly characteristically by means of her simple line technique. On a drawing at 6 ; 8, 20, we find three pictures of a girl with a broom. On one of these the girl has set the broom to the floor and is scrubbing with it. On the other she has just dipped it in a pail, and is holding it up so that the water drops off it ; in the third she is carelessly shaking the

[1] Lena Partridge, loc. cit., p. 175.
[2] Kerschensteiner, Die Entwicklung, etc., p. 34.
[3] F. Rosen, loc. cit., p. 15.

broom, so that the water is being sprinkled on tables and chairs. The motions are remarkably well observed and represented, although the arms are still simple lines, and the hand holding the broom a circular scribble.

Especially rapid progress in the drawing of posture and motion was reserved for Margaret's eighth year. She drew standing and sitting figures, also in back view ; the representation of a girl sitting at a piano with her back turned to the spectator is not successful, for the figure is standing in front of the piano-stool.   In " Karen's Birthday Party ", some of the little girls sitting on stools with their backs turned are comparatively correctly drawn.   She also began to draw figures bending down, for example, a little girl with a watering can bending over flowers to water them.   She was able to represent fairly truly, though formalized, the most various motions, persons walking, the pushing action of a person with a push-sleigh, running figures, and persons carrying out various actions.

Günther began at about the age of 5 to express movement. On one of his sea-pieces, a man is standing on a hill on the sea-shore and fishing.   On another, an Indian is holding a rope to which a diver is hanging. At 5 ; 6, he surprises us with a well-executed drawing of a monkey, hanging with both hands on to a ring and swinging.   The figure bending forward of St. Nicholas with his sack on his back, at 5 ; $8\frac{1}{2}$, is well observed and reproduced.   His drawing of a rider, at 6 ; 4, is not so good ; the fingers holding the reins are indicated, but the arm is missing and the foot, although in the stirrup, has no connection with the body.[1]

In the case of Walther-Heinz, we find only a few attempts during the first six years to represent motion. At 4 ; 8, we have a steersman holding the tiller of his ship ; at 5 ; 4, a captain shooting with a cannon ; at 5 ; 5, a locomotive driver holding the wheels of the steering apparatus ; the movement is everywhere given simply

[1] Stern, *loc. cit.*, pp. 13, 19, 24, 29.

by leading the lines of the arms to the point where they are supposed to be taking hold.[1]

Bubi's drawings, also, do not afford us many examples of the representation of motion. At 5½, Papa and Bubi are going out for a walk hand in hand, while Mama is waving from the window with a gigantic hand larger than her whole body. At 5 ; 9, he drew the Easter Hare running towards Bubi with a basket in its fore-paw, and a man rowing a boat with one oar, sitting sideways.[2]

Ekki, at 4 ; 7, drew "a man running", the fact being represented by the position of the legs ; at 4 ; 11, " Mama, Regina and Ekki dancing ", they are standing in a row and holding one another's hands. At 5 ; 2, a woman pushing a perambulator.[3]

Simonne drew, at the early age of 3 ; 4, 13, a lady carrying a basket, the fact being indicated by the lengthening of the arms towards the rounded form indicating the basket. This was an imitation of a drawing by her father having the same subject.[4] At 3 ; 7, 20, she said of a man drawn in a house, that he was " going out ", although this is in no way indicated by the drawing.[5] At about 5 ; 0, Simonne began to draw human figures, walking in the street, sitting at table, travelling in a carriage, without any indication in their posture or gestures. From the age of 5 ; 5 onwards, Simonne often pays attention in her drawing to actions. At 5 ; 5, 4, she drew a shop, with a lady going in and asking for a doll. She is turning to the shop-girl who appears here for the first time. She appears for the second time as going and fetching the doll, for the third time paying for the lady at the cash-desk, for the fourth time handing the lady the parcel with one hand and the change with the other. Finally, we see the lady in the street with the parcel in her hand.[6]

Luquet points out that the persons performing the

[1] Dix, loc. cit., pp. 85, 88, 89.
[2] Scupin, loc. cit., 2, pp. 190, 210, 258, 262.
[3] Krötzsch, loc. cit., p. 81.   [4] Luquet, loc. cit., p. 122, Fig. 39.
[5] loc. cit., p. 65, Fig. 368.   [6] loc. cit., p. 207, Fig. 879.

actions are represented in various positions, but the setting of the scene remains unchanged, and he reminds us that this is also to be seen in primitive folk-art. The place, the scenery, and everything which is unalterable, is only represented once, whereas the actors, and everything which changes, is repeated several times.[1] Rouma gives similar examples from children's drawings.[2] Rouma and F. Rosen also mention that similar cases are to be found in early Italian and Flemish paintings. Rosen refers to Ghirlandajo's picture of the "Adoration of the Shepherds in Bethlehem", where we see the procession of Wise Men from the East approaching along the road, and hence the events of the 24th of December, and the 6th of January, are shown on the same picture.[3]

Simonne's drawings, which were observed up to her ninth year, express movements and actions of the most various descriptions. Persons promenading, riding, driving, cycling, fishing, flying in an aeroplane, pushing a perambulator, carrying an umbrella, stick or basket, children playing, skipping, hitting a ball, etc. But her figures are always stiff and formalized, and the actions which are being carried out are usually represented by simple juxtaposition, by bringing the hand or the whole figure in contact with the object in question.

A seated figure does not appear; even at 8 ; 8, Simonne drew people, supposed to be sitting in a boat, horizontally across the seat, or more correctly under it, as the seat is visible across the figure.[4] Now and then, however, we find attempts to represent "partial, independent motions" (Rouma), arms bent or raised upwards, feet walking, etc.

Now and then a peculiar representation of motion appears in children's drawing. In Margaret's case this already appeared at 2 ; 0, 18. When she had finished her drawing of a flag, she made a quick stroke away from the flag and said: "There goes the flag." The

---

[1] Luquet, *loc. cit.*, p. 207, footnote.   [2] Rouma, *loc. cit.*, pp. 101 *et seq.*
[3] Rosen, *loc. cit.*, p. 23.   [4] Luquet, *loc. cit.*, Fig. 1663.

line was therefore intended to represent the motion in itself. Stern relates a similar fact of Günther at the age of 4. He wished to represent on a drawing, by closing a curtain, that darkness had come, and " passed his pencil over the paper with an energetic stroke from top to bottom as if he were pulling the cord of a curtain ". No misunderstanding was possible, it was not the cord itself, but the action of drawing it, which was to be expressed by the motion of the drawing pencil in a similar direction.[1] Miss Shinn tells us concerning her little niece Ruth that she drew a watch with a hand, and then said, " It goes round like that," drawing a circle to express the motion.[2] A fourteen-year-old boy represented the rapid motion of the screw on his aeroplane by drawing a dense mass of spiral lines.[3] Barnes reports of a boy that he represented " Johnny-Look-in-the-air " looking after the swallows by drawing a line from his eyes up to the swallows.[4] Rouma mentions similar observations.[5]

Parallels from folk-art can be found even for this comparatively rare characteristic of children's drawing. In the Härnevi Church in Uppland, for example, there is a fresco, in which we see, among other figures, a worldly man, apparently deep in prayer. His thoughts, however, are turned towards the goods of this world. In the picture, the path of his thoughts is shown by lines which issue from his mouth, one to his strong-box, others to his clothes, his well-appointed table, and his cask of wine.[6]

Otherwise, children's drawings and folk-art differ very greatly in their mode of representing movement. Understanding how to represent motion is above all things a matter of close observation and well-learned skill, and both of these are to be found only in a small degree in the case of children, but very highly developed in the

[1] Stern, *loc. cit.*, pp. 7, 9.   [2] Brown, *loc. cit.*, pp. 23 *et seq.*
[3] Rouma, *loc. cit.*, p. 104.
[4] Barnes, *A Study on Children's Drawings*, p. 460.
[5] Rouma, *loc. cit.*, p. 104.   [6] J. Ottosen, *Vor historie*, 2, p. 22.

case of savages. Hence the latter are often able to grasp and reproduce motion with astounding fidelity to nature. The oldest folk-art known to us, the palæolithic, begins, however, similarly to that of the child, with a formalized representation of animals, having only two stiff, stick-like legs without feet, devoid of any indication of motion.[1]

COLOUR

In works on the theory of art, laws such as " there are no such things as lines ", or " in the beginning was the coloured surface ", may be upheld. As regards children's drawing, the rule must read : " in the beginning was the line ". All children begin with lines and continue their drawing with colourless outline.

The biographies also show us that children in the early years, even when they have colours to hand, prefer to draw colourless outlines. Margaret had a red and blue pencil beside her, and watched me use them every day for drawing and colouring. But she usually took up an ordinary lead pencil to draw with, and only exceptionally did she scribble or draw outlines with red or blue. The only drawings really carried out in colour before she went to school are her ornament at the age of 4 ; 6, 3, her decorative flowers in red and blue at 5 ; 8, 20 and 5 ; 9, 6, and her flag drawings, at 6 ; 3. At first, she used colour, as do almost all children, for decorative purposes. Her first drawing in natural colour, or as Levinstein calls it, " local colour ", is her flag drawn from the model, and this was her only one before she went to school. Only when she was given coloured pencils at school and taught to use them, were her drawings coloured to a greater extent, but still only sparsely. Even in her seventh year, although she always had coloured pencils available, she usually made pencilled drawings when it was not a matter of a school drawing, and even when she coloured them, she only did it very sparingly. It was only in her eighth year that colour

[1] Hanna Rydh, *loc. cit.*, p. 130.

came into its own, and then she proceeded to carry out her free drawings with coloured pencils as a rule, more rarely with water-colours. For the most part she used colour naturalistically, as " local colour ", but now and then she also allowed herself some freedom in order to get a stronger decorative effect. Thus, she drew for preference green curtains which she had certainly never seen in reality ; curtains, dresses, and other materials are often represented in colours, these being the finest and most brilliant she could find, and put on in a peculiar stippling which she had invented herself (page 99). Altogether, her drawings of the eighth year bear witness to a sense of colour and a delight in it.

Simonne's drawings also were for a long time without colour, although from the time when, at the age of 3 ; 10, 12, she drew the outline of a man with red ink and blue pencil, she knew very well that she could find on her father's writing-table all that she needed for drawing red and blue lines. She only occasionally made coloured outlines. Her first representation of " local colour " is the scribbled indication of a blue sky at the age of 4 ; 8, 8. It was not until about her sixth year that she used colour and used it partly decoratively, partly naturalistically, and often in both ways in the same drawing.[1] For example, at 5 ; 4, 5, she drew a Tricolour, but not with equal strips of red, blue and white. Instead she put red in the middle, blue on both sides of it, and the white on the side most distant from the staff. At 5 ; 11, 3, she gave a flower realistic colours, made the roots brown, the leaves green, and the blossom yellow. At 7 ; 7, 20, she drew a lady, whose dress was decorated with colours, broad blue, brown, yellow, green, and rose-coloured stripes. In her hands the lady is carrying a basket, through which can be seen, in carefully chosen naturalistic colours, two green pears, a piece of rose-coloured meat, four red apples, four brown potatoes, two yellow oranges, and a red carrot with green leaves.[2]

[1] Luquet, *loc. cit.*, pp. 219 *et seq.*   [2] *loc. cit.*, pp. 219 *et seq.*

Stern reports that Günther already had in his fourth year great receptivity for colours and combination of colours. He noticed and admired spontaneously the play of coloured lights and colours in the landscape, in flowers, butterflies and so on. The activity of his interest in colour became particularly lively at the beginning of his sixth year. Besides chalk and lead pencil, the boy had coloured pencils available, which he used both to beautify his own productions as well as to fill in printed black and white outlines.[1] Walther-Heinz, to judge by the pictures reproduced, drew for the most part colourless outlines, although he too always had coloured pencils available. It is said of him at the age of 4 ; 4, that he coloured catalogue pictures industriously with coloured pencils. At 5 ; 4, he was given a box of water-colours, and then liked painting houses and trees with it, and colouring copies.[2] Bubi, although he is said to have had coloured pencils to hand, did not colour his drawings. Ekki does not seem to have used any colours for drawing.

From the biographical studies, therefore, it must be concluded that children, in their first five or six years, prefer to represent the general form of objects by colourless outlines. At about the age of six they begin to carry out their drawings in colour more frequently.

As regards school-children, according to Levinstein's observations they prefer to draw with coloured pencil and water-colours when they can get them. Only a few children then prefer lead pencil. The outline is drawn in lead pencil and filled in with colour.[3]

The first use of colour is made in a formalized and decorative manner. Outlines are filled with strong colour without reference to the actual appearance of the object. Naturalistic colours can, however, already be found in the formula period, objects being given in the natural local colour, the colour corresponding to the real appear-

[1] Stern, *loc. cit.*, pp. 17, 30. [2] Dix, *loc. cit.*, pp. 68, 83, 87.
[3] Levinstein, *loc. cit.*, pp. 31, 32.

ance of the object seen from close to. A tree-trunk is painted brown, the leaves green, and so on. It is only very late, and rarely without being told, that the child goes so far as to represent natural colours and colour perspective.[1]

The most ancient folk-art begins, like that of a child, with lines and outlines. The earliest known cave pictures are outline drawings, the lines of which are engraved or drawn in red or black colour. Here, as in the drawing of children, the lines are first painted, and only later is the surface inside the outline coloured. " The colour which begins close to the thick outline, is spread more and more over the whole figure of the animal. Sometimes the whole body of the animal is hatched in colour, and later fully painted." [2] The next colour period also of children's drawing finds its parallels in early folk-art. Colour is used, as by the child, to paint in surfaces in single colours within the outline, and is then as in the child's case, " local colour " without light and shade or atmospheric perspective. Examples of this are found in palæolithic, Assyrian and Egyptian art, in Greek Vase painting, in the Middle Ages, and to some extent also in the art of the early Renaissance.[3]

ORNAMENT

It is a quite general observation that we seek in vain in the earliest drawings of children for genuine, self-invented ornament. Narrative drawing appears, according to all observations, earlier than decorative, which, as Bühler thinks, usually occupies a place only after the sixth year.[4] Sully already draws attention to the feeble development of the æsthetic sense in children.[5] Dix found no ornaments in his son's drawings of the first six years ; we can scarcely follow Dix in speaking of decorative drawing when a flag or flowers are shown

---

[1] Levinstein, *loc. cit.*, p. 32.
[2] Hanna Rydh, *loc. cit.*, pp. 129 *et seq.*
[3] Rosen, *loc. cit.*, pp. 7 *et seq.*
[4] Bühler, *loc. cit.*, pp. 139, 140.   [5] Sully, *loc. cit.*, p. 318.

on a balcony in colours.[1] Günther and Bubi, too, took no interest in ornament in the first six years, while Ekki,

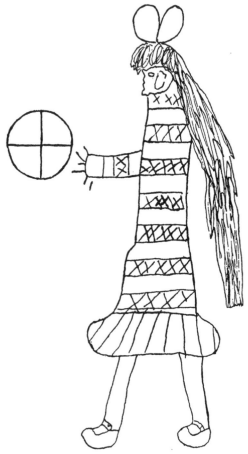

FIG. 131.—GIRL PLAYING BALL. MARGARET, 7 ; 10, 15. ORIGINAL IN COLOURS. DRESS AND HAIR-RIBBON BLUE, BALLS RED, YELLOW, GREEN AND BLUE. 1/1.

who was gifted with an unusual sense of rhythm, already put zig-zag lines around his drawing for decoration at

[1] Dix, *loc. cit.*, p. 95.

the age of three. He later showed an interest for ornament unusual with children ; he drew dots, circles,
ovals, zig-zag and wavy lines as frame or decoration
for writing and pictures. Now and then he produced
patterns—circles divided by lines with dots in the spaces,
a coverlet with flower ornament, and so on.[1] Simonne
now and then also produced line patterns, for the only
reason " that they are pretty ", but Luquet points out
that attempts at ornament in Simonne's drawings only
appear in very limited number and quite ephemerally.[2]
We find in Margaret's drawings primitive ornament at
4 ; 6, 3, produced by drawing, " in order to make it
pretty ", parts of a line of equal length alternately with
red and blue pencil. At 6 ; 3, 1, and 6 ; 4, 28, she
drew strips of trimming for dresses. In the eighth

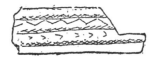

FIG. 132.—PIECE OF BONE WITH ORNAMENT. FROM LAUGERIE-
BASSE, DORDOGNE. OLD STONE AGE. (FROM REINACH.)

year she gave dresses patterned edgings or, more frequently, patterns consisting of coloured dots. An
example for this is seen in her " girl playing ball " at
7 ; 10, 15 (Fig. 131). The pattern on the dress is simple
and invented by herself ; but similar cross-patterns, and
also zig-zag lines and other simple geometrical ornaments,
are often found in primitive folk-art (Fig. 132). Margaret's doors, staircases and garden fences were also
decorated with various patterns. Her picture " the
Queen and the Court Ladies ", at about 7 ; 10, 15, shows
a peculiar attempt at decorative art ; the little figures
placed on each side of the door and above the lintel
are there " to make it grand ", the door and the window
have a more stately form than in ordinary houses, and

[1] Krötzsch, loc. cit., pp. 19 et seq., 35 et seq.
[2] Luquet, loc. cit., pp. 166 et seq.

the chairs of the Court Ladies are decorated with balls. Similar little figures were used in one of Margaret's drawings at about this time to decorate the frame of a mirror.

Bühler points out, that one can well imagine theoretically a transition from scribbling to ornament alongside the usual transition from scribbling to representation. " If the beginnings of scribbling are really practised as we have assumed, from motor pleasure in play, the transition from this to the most primitive ornamental drawings may be called but a short step. Fundamentally, nothing more is necessary at the beginning than a direction of interest and play pleasure to the products of this activity, to the lines themselves." [1] Bühler takes the concept of graphical ornament in its very widest sense, " so that all graphic forms, which either have no function as drawing, or at least have not been produced for its sake, are to be included in the concept." [2]

The interest in lines for their own sake and the pleasure in playing with lines was, according to my observation, a chief motive for Margaret's attempts to draw, from the very first stroke that she made. According to Bühler's definition, therefore, her whole scribbling consisted of ornament. His definition appears to me to be a little too comprehensive ; in any case, one must certainly add to it, that the elements of form are to occur in rhythmic repetition, or to fill a space, and have been produced " to make it pretty ". Even with this limitation, certain of Margaret's scribbles might almost be pronounced to be ornaments, as when she filled a sheet of paper with long and regular zig-zag or spiral lines, or drew equally long pieces of zig-zag lines alternatively with red and blue pencil. In any case, the unquestionable primitive ornament at 4 ; 6, 3, arose directly out of her scribbling.

I made this observation in the case of another girl. At 4 ; 3, she drew a little girl in a fairly well developed

[1] Bühler, *loc. cit.*, p. 138.   [2] *loc. cit.*, p. 138.

formalized manner. Thereupon she scribbled zig-zag lines right across the whole dress and around it and explained that this was " *Nann* ", that is to say, *name*, which again means the same as writing. " Like you write it in the book," she said, " it's to make it grand." Here again we meet with primitive ornament, which likewise has the meaning of writing. It is just this kind of scribble, really only a shortened and vertical wavy scribble, that develops in Margaret's drawing gradually into the first real writing. Ornament as well as writing can therefore develop, in the child's drawing directly from scribbling as a common origin.

Bühler observes in connection with his above-mentioned theory, that the ornament of primitive races might have developed directly from a play with lines similar to children's scribbling, or also from lines and form-elements produced by chance during the work of making useful objects, from the scratches produced in rock during the grinding of a stone axe, from lines scratched with a knife in wood, from finger-prints in clay, during modelling, and so on.[1] Whether representative drawing, or ornament, is the original form of the art of primitive races, is a very controversial question. Some investigators have maintained that all ornaments arose from the stylized drawing of objects or motives from nature. It has been pointed out that representative drawing, and above all highly skilful representation of animals, was pre-eminent in palæolithic times ; ornament, on the other hand, in the subsequent neolithic period.   T. Wilson rejects this theory and draws attention to the presence of geometric ornament in palæolithic art as well.   It consisted of parallel lines, sometimes crossed, sometimes running in various directional zig-zag lines, x-shaped lines, wavy lines, and similar geometrical patterns. He maintains that palæolithic models were repeated again and again in the Neolithic and Bronze Age ; they were varied and developed further, but up to the end of the

[1] Bühler, *loc. cit.*, p. 139.

prehistoric period and beginning of the historic, no advance was made beyond simple geometrical ornament.[1] Later investigators have also shown that purely geometrical ornaments arise independently in the earliest art, and are to be found alongside pictorial representation ; but ornament may also, but much more rarely, be developed by stylization.[2]

[1] T. Wilson, *The Prehistoric Art*, pp. 412, 418, 419.
[2] Hoernes-Menghin, *Urgeschichte dei bildenden Kunst in Europa*, pp. 28 *et seq.*, 574, 654, 194, 195.

CHILDREN'S DRAWING AS AN EXPRESSION OF THEIR MENTAL DEVELOPMENT

FROM the point of view of psychology, the study of children's drawing has quite particular interest. An uninterrupted series of a child's spontaneous drawings gives, as it were, a psychographic representation of the growth of the child's mind during the time when it was still developing freely and naturally, without any kind of compulsions from school or instruction. It may be objected, it is true, that the mental process behind the child's drawing is a special and peculiar one, so that no conclusion can be arrived at concerning general mental development from an examination of the drawing. The fact that this objection does not hold good is shown by the wide parallelism that can be proved to exist between the child's drawing and its speech, its formation of concepts and its thinking.

Just as the child commences its drawing with a meaningless scribble of useless lines and forms endlessly repeated, so speech begins with meaningless and repeated babbling of sounds and syllables. The scribbling period in the child's drawing corresponds to the babbling in its talk. Both for drawing and speech, the child at first can find only formalized expressions. Just as the child indicates a human figure by means of a simple formalized outline, a circle, so does it express the whole sense of a sentence such as " I want to sit on Mother's knee " by the single word " Mother ". It enlarges its human formula with a new characteristic : two lines as legs—it adds to its sentence formula a new word : " Mother sit ". Just as the child draws single persons and objects fragmentally and without connection, so it places single principal sentences in loose connection one beside the other. It gradually enriches its drawings with new detailism and adds to them situations and landscapes ; it enlarges its sentences with new parts of sentences and word forms, and connects them by various conjunctions, but a child's language, like its drawing, has a formalized character, taken as a whole, even into the school age.

Many parallels may also be found between the child's drawing and its formation of concepts. Just as a child's first concepts are primal concepts, which comprehend in the same word a series of different things, so also we may say that it uses primal formulæ in its drawing, a formula for all animals, one for all sorts of trees, and so on. Primal concept and primal formula have both too large a scope and too little content, they are badly defined and poor in points of differentiation. The primal formula, like the primal concept, also gradually differentiates itself, it gains a distinctive content and is correctly limited. The child's first concepts are often uncertain, they appear and disappear again, and the same is true in its drawing. It acquires a fairly good human formula, but is not able to retain it, so it degenerates into scribbling. A second formula appears and disappears, and so on. At times it gives its human figures hair, teeth, ears and other features, which are omitted again after a short time. Investigations concerning the child's formation of concepts have shown that it acquires, as a rule, certain general and comprehensive concepts, such as trees, flowers, before it has learned to distinguish single trees and single flowers, just as in drawing it expresses all trees and all flowers by the same formula. This does not mean to say that the child has formed comprehensive logical general concepts, but rather that it is deficient in experience, and in capacity for correct analysis and synthesis. In a given case, " flower " may be applied also to a tree on account of chance points of likeness, or the other way round, just as a child when drawing often uses the same formula, a circular scribble and a straight line, to indicate a tree or a flower. Conversely it also happens that the child's formula represents no generally comprehensive concept, but is limited to a single definite mental picture. Thus Margaret's first human formula does not stand for the human figure generally ; she sees only Mama or sometimes Margaret herself in it. In the same way also, the child's concepts are often limited to single definite individual ideas. The child's concepts are at first poor, and later richer, in content, like its formalized drawings. In children's drawing, as in children's thinking, a characteristic want of connection is revealed. Just as the child when drawing places objects in a row, detached, and without deeper and closer relation, so the placing side by side of concepts is one of the most general characteristics of its thinking. The want of power of abstraction, of penetrating analysis, of richer or more manifold synthesis appear both in the drawing and in the thinking of a child.[1]

In drawing, as in the child's power of forming images, progress is found to be from simple mental images to compound, from the formalized and incomplete to one more true to appearances, from the general and indefinite and the individually indefinite through intermediate stages to the more definite, from the few to the many, from the isolated to the connected, from chance connections to those dominated by a leading idea.

The development of children's drawing before the school years, assuming that they are given no teaching or other direct influence, may be regarded as an example of a natural process of learning. Spontaneous drawing teaches us how a child, growing up in civilized life, learns something by itself, how it unfolds its powers, what it takes from its surroundings and what it seeks and takes from other persons, who of course should not force anything upon it.

[1] Cf. Helga Eng, *Abstrakte Begriffe im Sprechen und Denken des Kindes.*

If we consider children's drawing as expression of a natural process of learning, we find that its chief characteristics can be described as imitation and self-expression, repetition and new acquisitions.

All investigators have found that the beginnings of children's drawing depend upon imitation, and that imitation also plays an important part in its further development in this respect. The child copies the drawings of others and its own drawings, it imitates its mental pictures of objects and its mental pictures of the pictures of objects. It imitates the drawing movements of others, and when drawing its own movements. The use of the materials and means is also imitation.

A copy acts on well-endowed children not only as a motive for repeating it, but likewise as a spur to self-expression. The child's scribbling is spontaneous, for it has never seen a model for this peculiar wavy scribbling. The development of its scribbling is an unfolding of itself, although imitation may play a certain part, for example, as in the transition to circular scribbling. The various phases are passed through without any interference from its environment. When a child puts a circle and two lines together and calls this " Mama ", we meet with a creative act, although imitation plays its part. Without being asked or instructed, and without having seen others drawing, the child develops its art over a period of years, it practises voluntarily, takes up new motives, commences to " compose " pictures, acquires the most important points of perspective representation, and so on. The child teaches itself of its own free will. The child does not take impressions from its environment passively ; it makes a selection and works them over, and when they again appear represented in its drawing, they bear the impress of the child's mind. We are dealing here not only with imitation but with self-expression.

Repetition and novelty are the two other main characteristics in the development of the child's drawing. It repeats its wavy scribble endlessly in the first few months ; it acquires new forms of scribble and repeats them a hundred times ; in the same way it repeats its formalized drawings. At the beginning, so long as the child only has a few motives and practised forms of drawing, repetition plays the greater part ; then new motives begin to appear continually, and are repeated. They gradually become more complete by repetition, and acquire new detail ; even older children still repeat their drawings, although not so often as when younger, perhaps only three, four or five up till ten or twelve times. The child thus gradually devotes more time to the acquirement and execution of new motives, and less time to repetition, which, however, still sometimes plays an important part, also in the form of free scribbling practice. Repetitions serve to practise the act of drawing, which can then be performed more quickly, and economy of energy takes place, which is applied to new progress, the mastery of new motives or new details.

A curious phenomenon, which much surprises the observer, is the apparently planned and purposeful practice, even in the child's first years of life. Margaret practised circles and straight lines and drew her first human formula at 1 ; 10 ; she practised angles and rectangles and reached her goal of drawing a tram. I observed the same trait in her linguistic development ; when, for example, she had just acquired the use of the perfect and imperfect, she endeavoured to make use of these continually when speaking, so that one got the impression of intentional practice. Other biographies also indicate that the little artists are given to practising. In the earliest years practice and repetition are no doubt for the most part ideomotive, the mental picture of the movement produces the movement. Later on the latter is gradually carried out more consciously and independently. At 6 ; 4, 28, Margaret answered my question, as to how she had learnt to draw a certain motive, by saying " I practised it." It is altogether not unlikely that we should find with more careful study that little children observe and learn more consciously than we are inclined to suppose.

The child takes impressions from its environment; pictures and picture-books give it motives and models for its representation, the impulse comes to it from observing how others draw and write; it asks others to draw something for it, asks all sorts of questions about matters connected with its practice, in other words, it gets instruction through its own initiative.

Although the child, therefore, imbibes a great deal from its surroundings, its drawing is nevertheless unquestionably the spontaneous unfolding of an inner bent. The influence of environment was shown by Ruth Griffiths's experiments. She collected and studied drawings by two groups of children of pre-school age. The children in one group lived in crowded tenements in one, of the poorest districts in London, and the other similar group of children was from Brisbane in Australia. The Australian children were from good homes, most of them had gardens, where the children were among trees, flowers and birds continually. They lived a healthy life in the open air and in close contact with nature, they visited the country and the seaside. It is stated that it would be difficult to find more different environmental conditions. Other factors were kept constant in the experiment, e.g. the intelligence quotients were similar in both groups, though they varied from child to child within each group.

The results show clearly the influence of the milieu. The Brisbane children made more than double the number of drawings, they talked more about them and used more colour. There was, however, no essential difference between the two groups with respect to the quality of the drawing. This shows that the drawing is also determined by inner factors which are more alike in the two groups and more independent of environment.[1]

By a penetrating analysis Ruth Griffiths found eleven stages of evolution in the drawings of these children. These stages were regularly, though not simultaneously

[1]Ruth Griffiths, *Imagination in Early Childhood*, pp. 344, 347 *et seq.*

gone through by all children in both groups.[1] This finding suggests that the development of children's spontaneous drawing depends on the maturation of psychic traits which are essentially determined by heredity and are relatively independent of their environments.

One of these psychic traits is intelligence, and Ruth Griffiths states on the basis of her experiments that there is a high correlation between mental age and development of drawing and demonstrates it graphically.[2] This was corroborated by Florence Goodenough, who has worked out a measuring scale of intelligence for children on the basis of the drawing of a man. This test correlates 0.763 with the Stanford-Binet intelligence test.[3] The IQ on the drawing test is determined by the completeness of the child's representation of the traits of the man's figure and the details in his dress.[4]

The child's drawings witness to the development of its power of attention, which at first is not able to hold fast the mental pictures or to direct movement, but then becomes firmer, more comprehensive, and more intentional. The drawing indicates how the child's power of observation and analysis develop, its capacity for synthesis, thinking and power of judgment grow.

The child's drawings testify to an imagination which is active and lively, although weak and planless. It ascribes sensible interpretations to the figures it produces with unhesitating daring and only the slightest indication of likeness. It flits in chance associations from idea to idea, with only a slight hold on objective reality. Later on the child's imagination becomes gradually more able to follow a leading idea and to create an organic whole in its drawings.

The child's spontaneous drawings reflect is feelings and interests. They tell us what it has at heart and what it finds meaningful and interesting. Even if the child's drawings seem stiff and lifeless in the eyes of the adult they may nevertheless be the expression of emotions to

[1]*loc. cit.*, pp 209 *et seq.*   [2]*loc. cit.*, p. 212.
[3]Florence Goodenough, *Measurement of Intelligence by Drawings*.
[4]This favours the boys, who more often draw a man. The girls ought to be allowed to draw a girl or a " lady ".

the child himself. They show the child's aesthetic feelings and interests. Children are in the early years more interested in form and less in colour. This was corroborated by the results of an investigation by P. Engel. He found that of children under $3\frac{1}{2}$ years 90 per cent show more (passive) interest in form, 5 per cent in colour. He ascribes to this fact a biological meaning. Among the children $3\frac{1}{2}$—6 years 86.6 per cent were more interested (passively) in colour, 13.3 per cent more in form[1]. After that age the passive interest in form again increases. Biographical studies show, in confirmation, that active use of colour begins about the age of six, and develops with increasing age. The child's sense of form develops, so that the formless and disproportioned figures and forms of the early years gradually become somewhat better shaped. The child may early show some interest in rhythm, harmony and proportion, as when Margaret fills a sheet of paper with scribbled lines and tries to have like space in between (31, 34, 38). Most of Margaret's drawings have a harmonious picture order, especially in later years. She may even intuitively make use of aesthetic measures. In " Court Ladies " (106) the picture order is in the main strictly symmetrical, and the side-lines of the door frame build golden sections with the opposite outer lines. " St. Hanshaugen " (111) has a harmonious picture order and golden sections horizontally and vertically, etc.

Children's drawings reflect the growth of will and activity from simple, automatic meaningless movements to compound, intentional, planned actions.

Essential psychic processes are active in the child's spontaneous drawing, not in isolation, but integrated in the whole organic psychic activity. A study of the child's drawing may, therefore, help to understand its individual character, its problems and special needs.

The evolution of the child's free, spontaneous drawing is the expression of the development of the child's personality.

[1] P. Engel, *Uber die inhaltliche Beachtung von Farbe und Form*, pp. 210, 212, 243, 250.

CHILDREN'S DRAWING AND FOLK-ART.

IF we compare children's drawing and folk-art, we must first consider the oldest graphic art known to us. This belongs to palæolithic times (the Old Stone Age), and its traces have been mainly found in the caves of France and Spain. The men of the Old Stone Age were hunters and fishermen; they had no fixed dwellings and were probably at a very primitive stage of mental development. But on the walls and ceilings of the caves which served them as dwelling-places, on bones and horns of animals slain by them, artistic representations have been found of such vivacity and truth to nature, that they cannot but excite the greatest admiration (Figs. 133 and 134). The art of the child is first concerned with the representation of the human figure, folk-art with the representation of animals.[1]

In palæolithic pictures we find animals living at the time, mammoths, bison, reindeer, horses, ibex, and so on, and sometimes sea animals, such as seals, sea-lions and fishes, and also a few birds.[2] Human beings are rarely, and not so well represented.

The engraving and painting on rock walls in Northern countries, of the Old Stone Age period, are of the same nature of palæolithic art. They likewise show mostly animals, particularly reindeer and elk, and in the same lively and characteristic fashion (Fig. 135).[3]

---

[1] If we include the art of sculpture, folk-art really begins with the human figure, for a few little statuettes have been found belonging to the early Aurignac period—mostly female figures—which are taken to be the first start of artistic production.

[2] S. Reinach, *Repertoire de l'Art quaternaire.* Hoernes-Menghin, *loc. cit.*, pp. 116 *et seq.*

[3] G. Hallström, "Hällristningar i norra Skandinavien", *Ymer*, 27, 1907, and "Nordskandinaviska hällristningar", *Fornvännen*, 2, 3, 4, 1907–1909.

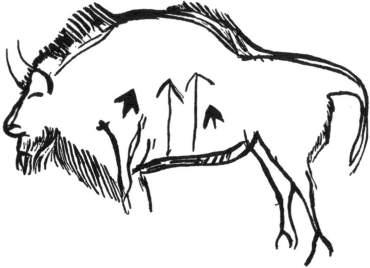

FIG. 133.—DRAWING ON CAVE WALL IN BLACK OUTLINE, FROM THE
"BLACK SALON" AT NIAUX ARIEGE. BISON. SEVERAL ARROWS,
TWO OF WHICH ARE RED, ARE POINTING AT IT. (FROM CARTAILHAC
AND BREUIL.) REPRODUCED FROM HANNA RYDH.

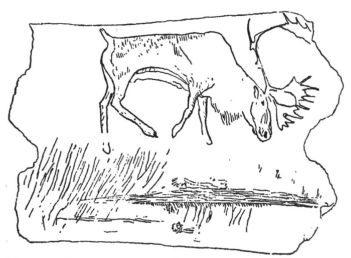

FIG. 134.—REINDEER GRAZING. ENGRAVED ON REINDEER HORN IN
THE OLD STONE AGE. FOUND IN THE KESSLERLOCH IN THAY-
INGEN, SWITZERLAND. 2/3. (FROM WILSON.)

H. Shetelig thinks that the twin art-forms are so essentially similar that it is difficult to imagine that they arose independently of one another ; the only logically satisfactory explanation would be that this art was carried to Northern Europe while still living, in the latest palæolithic period, in Western Europe.[1]

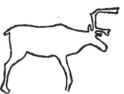

In the Neolithic and Bronze Ages, great changes took place in human life and art. Mankind ceased to be nomad, tilled the soil, kept domestic animals and carried on industry. Religious and metaphysical notions came into existence. Art consisted in

FIG. 135.—ENGRAVING FROM THE STONE AGE. DRAWING OF A REINDEER BY THE BROOK BOLA IN STOD, NORTHERN NORWAY. (FROM G. HALLSTRÖM.)

abstract geometrical ornament, used to decorate clay vessels, utensils, weapons and jewellery. We rarely meet with attempts to represent animals, human beings, or natural objects of any kind.[2]

A naturalistic art similar to the Palæolithic is found among several primitive races at the present day, for example, the Bushmen (Fig. 136), the Eskimos, a few Indian tribes (Fig. 137) ; while on the other hand, many present-day savages are at a lower level in the matter of artistic representation.

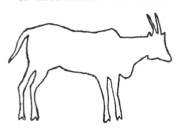

FIG. 136.—ENGRAVING MADE BY BUSHMEN ON A CLIFF. (FROM FRITSCH AND GROSSE.)

As has been shown by several examples, children's drawings have many features in common with primitive folk-art. No one can deny the correctness of this observation, but how far this

---

[1] H. Shetelig, " Norsk kunst i de eldste tider ", Norsk kunsthistorie, p. 14.
[2] Hoernes-Menghin, loc. cit., pp. 192 et seq.

parallelism goes, what its inward and outward causes are, and what conclusions may be drawn from it, are all controversial questions, and opinions are very much divided.

In the affirmation of this parallelism, and in drawing bold conclusions from it, probably the one to go farthest is the German historian Lamprecht : " Three roads to further advance in human psychogenesis are open to us ; the history of civilization, ethnography, and · child psychology."

Of these three sciences, that of the history of civilization is the easiest to apply, since it has a comparatively trustworthy chronology.

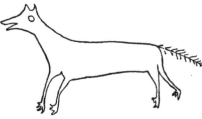

FIG. 137.—PRAIRIE WOLF DRAWN BY A KOOTENAY INDIAN. (FROM CHAMBERLAIN.)

The case of ethnography is otherwise. The numerous facts are usually not available in chronological order, and if we consider the development of various races at a low level of culture, no single means is known of finding out which of these races, relatively to the others, has progressed farthest or remained most backward. Here it appears to me that something could be done by means of child psychology. It is certain that the child's mental development, at least in Europe and North America, passes through the same phases, and I believe we may regard it as certain that these phases will be found in the case of children all over the world. Some of these periods, particularly the more advanced, agree with the various stages of development known to us from ethnology, or parallel with them. If we gain a knowledge of the phases of the child's psychical development, it should be possible to apply the chronological results of child psychology to the ethnographic data, to "historicize " them, so to speak.

Apart from this first noteworthy service which child psychology can render to history, there is still another. By its aid we might learn those phases of human psychogenesis for which ethnographic sources are either entirely wanting, or insufficient.

"Clearly we ought to pay especial attention to the sources of child psychology most nearly corresponding to primitive historical sources. I am thinking, in the first place, of modelling and drawing." "A systematic study of children's drawing would be of great use to us." [1]

Rouma, as one of Lamprecht's collaborators in collecting children's drawings in large numbers, became aware that Lamprecht's method gave scope for many mistakes and erroneous interpretations. This led him to concern himself with the comparative study of children's drawings and folk-art, and he was led to the result that the great similarity between the two is more apparent than real. He points out that no present-day child, or adult of average ability, could produce drawings fit to compare with the art of the Stone Age, of the Bushmen, or of the Eskimos. On the other hand, it has been found that drawings collected by explorers and carried out at their request by average persons of savage peoples, are crude and formal, and in many ways like those of our own children : for example, the Koch-Grünberg drawings made by the Indians of Central Brazil. Rouma thinks that this is to be explained by the drawings preserved from palæolithic times having been executed, not by average persons, but by those of unusual artistic powers. These probably attained their high level, basing upon artistic tradition and construction, by practice ; we find their sketches and designs in the caves which they inhabited. The case of the Bushmen is similar, and the Eskimos, as we know, practise from early childhood. Their pictorial representations are

<hr>

[1] K. Lamprecht, " Les dessins d'enfants comme source historique ", Communication and lecture, *Bull. de l'Académie royale de Belgique* (*classe des lettres, etc.*), 9–10, pp. 461 *et seq.*, 1906.

made by specialists, and hence cannot be compared with the products of an average primitive man unpractised in drawing, nor with those of average children, who draw because they see others drawing, or because they are put to it at school or in the Kindergarten.

If we were to proceed to a classification as proposed by Lamprecht, it would lead us to assign a higher position to races at a lower level, such as men of the Stone Age, the Bushmen, and the Eskimos; while races actually at a more advanced cultural stage, practising agriculture, living in settlements, keeping domestic animals, engaged in industry, and having acquired metaphysical and abstract ideas, would be placed in a lower position as being less skilful artists.

The primitive races which produce the best art are hunters, who have practised their visual and manual powers from childhood. The child's drawings at the first stage bear the stamp of its visual and manual inability. If we try to compare here the products of graphic art, great differences are certain to appear.

Similarities are only likely to be found in those aspects of drawing which depend upon the power of voluntary attention and abstraction. The work in both cases is always concrete, and if the understanding of perspective representation is brought into the comparison, insuperable difficulties are met with.

Rouma concludes that the artistic work of primitive races is so dependent upon environment, occupation, metaphysical ideas, and so forth, that a comparison with children's drawings is impossible, and further, that the artistic production of a race cannot provide a sufficient foundation for the assessment of its level of culture.[1]

M. Verworn attempts to explain the development of primitive art by a peculiar theory. The high-grade naturalistic art of the palæolithic period he calls *physioplastic*, that of the neolithic and Bronze Age, *ideoplastic*; the latter was formalized and abstract, and consisted

---

[1] Rouma, *loc. cit.*, pp. 243 *et seq.*

mainly of geometrical ornament. Verworn sees the cause of the transition from physioplastic to ideoplastic art in the idea of the soul. Starting from the idea of the soul, a quantity of religious ideas are developed, which soon rule the life of primitive races. " This stage of naïve theorizing, and weird and bizarre products of the imagination, corresponds to ideoplastic art." [1]

As far as we know, thinks Verworn, the palæolithic hunter had no ideas of the soul and all connected therewith. He did not think about such things at all. He did not seek for anything behind phenomena. He knew nothing of metaphysics. He reckoned with what he saw. He was similar in every way to the Bushman. [2]

We can find the same among savage tribes at the present time. All races, the whole life of which is ruled by religious ideas and notions of the soul, such as the Negroes, Indians, islanders of the Indian Ocean, have an ideoplastic art in an extreme degree. But in the case of the Bushmen, so long as they do not come into contact with more cultivated neighbours, religious ideas are, it would seem, entirely wanting. The art of the Bushmen is almost exclusively physioplastic. [3]

The prehistoric and ethnographical facts thus lead to the same conclusions as physiological and psychological analysis—primitive art is physioplastic in the measure of a preponderant development of sense impressions ; it is ideoplastic to the extent to which the life of abstract and theoretical ideas has reached a higher development. [4] Art becomes divorced from reality, because along with theorizing and reflection concerning man and his environment, an overdevelopment of the imagination, not so much of the memory, commences. This overplus of ideas, thinks Verworn, leads by psychological necessity to the single images becoming abstract. In a later work, Verworn sees the foundations of ideoplastic art less in the overabundance of ideas, than in increasing abstraction. [5]

---

[1] Verworn, *Zur Psychologie der primitiven Kunst*, p. 726.
[2] *loc. cit.*, p. 726. [3] *loc. cit.*, p. 727.
[4] *loc. cit.*, p. 727. [5] Verworn, *Ideoplastische Kunst*.

Verworn concludes that the child's art cannot, as one might have expected from biogenetic law, be regarded as parallel with the physioplastic art of palæolithic times, but rather with the strictly ideoplastic art of the later age.[1]

As we shall see later, Verworn's theory as applied to palæolithic art cannot be correct, but it may still hold good for the transition from palæolithic to neolithic art.

Bühler objects that painters would be in a bad way if an abundance of ideas stood in the way of true representation. Most of the really great ones had, as a rule, an excess of mental images, and many of them painted chiefly from memory. Bühler points out that it is not at all necessary that such imaginative pictures be formalized and stylized, since there exists, alongside the imaginative power which stylizes, one which is true to appearances, and is psychologically more fundamental. Formalized drawing might arise without animism, and this is shown by children's drawing, for no one would seek in them the expression of an animistic way of thinking.

Bühler, however, considers that Verworn is right in seeking for the cause of the transition from physioplastic to ideoplastic art in changes in the imaginative point of view, which in the case of drawing from memory plays as important a part as observation. It is not sufficient to point out that primitive races whose art is physioplastic are hunters, with acute senses and great manual skill ; other hunter races exist with a highly developed power of observation and manual dexterity, whose pictorial representations are quite as formalized and undeveloped as those of children. Bühler is inclined to ascribe to language and conceptual thinking a similar influence to that ascribed by Verworn to animism. Bühler considers the possibility that little children have at first mental pictures true to nature, but that they then become formalized and abstract under the influence

---

[1] Verworn, *Zur Psychologie, etc.*, p. 724.

of language.[1] In the section on the formalized drawing of children I have endeavoured to show that this cannot be the case, since the child's imaginative life, and its speech, its drawing and other mental processes, are to begin with formalized and incomplete, and gradually develop greater perfection and truth to nature. The most ancient folk-art shows, as we shall see later, the same development.

A kernel of truth may lie in the views of Verworn and Bühler. Even if Verworn lays too great a stress on the awakening of the idea of the soul, it is not improbable that a growing abundance of metaphysical and abstract ideas, of conceptual speaking and thinking, may contribute towards making artistic forms of expression more abstract and less naturalistic. But it can only be a matter of a contributive, not a sole cause, for otherwise all folk-art would tend to become more formalized with increasing mental development, and the same would be true of children's drawing, which should become more formalized with increase of age and growth of the power of abstract thought. But this is not the case. Nevertheless, it would not be unthinkable that impulses from the environment and an inherited capacity for abstract and conceptual thought might play a part and favour the formalized style in the child's drawing. A contribution to the decision of this question would be gained by investigating whether children's drawing among races having a high-grade naturalistic art, for example the Eskimos, is less formalized. Available investigations on this point are not sufficient, but there are certain observations which suggest a confirmation. Chamberlain reports the judgment given by Louisa McDermott concerning seven hundred and twenty drawings of Indian children : " Indian children have a greater inborn talent for drawing than white children ; they also develop earlier. This is shown in a better control over the motions of the hand." Marguerite Gallagher

[1] Bühler, *loc. cit.*, pp. 181 *et seq.*

says concerning three hundred freely executed drawings of Indian children compared with those of white children at the same age : " Their drawings have a greater content of life. There are more stories told in a corresponding number of other drawings." [1] Louise Maitland obtained from a member of an Alaska expedition sixty-five drawings of Eskimo boys and girls under fourteen years of age ; some of them had attended a school for several years, but none of them could read or write English. She says of these drawings that they showed a highly developed power of observation, for without it they could not be so characteristic. " Everything in these drawings is full of life and motion. At the same time, we find the mistakes characteristic of children's drawings, mixed profiles, confusion of plan and elevation, transparency, turning over."

These observations are corroborated by a more systematic investigation which was recently carried out by R. J. Havighurst, M. K. Gunther and J. E. Pratt. They administered Goodenough's drawing test to 325 Indian children. The result was that the IQ of these Indian children were 110—117 on the drawing test; their drawings of a man were of a higher quality than the drawings of white American children. The reason according to the interpretation of the authors, is that Indian children have more opportunity of observing different motifs, and the human figure.

To judge by all available material, palæolithic artists must have worked from memory, but here also opinions are divided. Wilson thinks that they worked from the model.[2] Wundt assumes that their drawing in the dim caves in which they lived must have been made from memory. " At the primitive stage only art from memory exists." [3] Primitive lamps, such as those found in the la Mouthe Cave, could certainly not have supplied a

[1] Chamberlain, *loc. cit.*, p. 197.
[2] Wilson, *loc. cit.*, p. 412.
[3] W. Wundt, *Elemente der Völkerspychologie*, pp. 24, 25, 107.

very bright light.[1] To produce such an art from memory the people of the Palæolithic Age must have had unusually intense visual images. Jaensch therefore supposes them to have possessed similar " eidetic " gifts to those found in the case of youth. The " eidetics " have mental pictures intermediate between imagination and perception, and these pictures may be quite as lively and definite as direct vision. Jaensch bases his view on the material collected by Lévy-Bruhl in his book, *Les fonctions mentales dans les sociétés inférieures*, and thinks that " it compels us to draw the conclusion that the sensual and imaginative world of savages is very close to the eidetic world of youth ".[2]

In more recent years the relation between eidetic and drawing has been investigated by a number of psychologists. P. Metz states on the basis of experiments that the eidetic image is of no direct use in the act of drawing.

The drawing of the average child can certainly not compare with that of adult primitive man, in spite of all points of contact. In looking through a book containing drawings of both, for example Levinstein's, one can in most cases decide at the first glance whether a drawing originated from primitive folk-art or a present-day child. It has been asserted that primitive folk-art is on the same level as the drawing of the *gifted* child. But if we investigate the reproductions of gifted children's drawings in Kik's and Hartlaub's studies, we find that the drawings of children, as long as they draw *as* children, always show, in spite of all their good points, signs of formalism, stiffness, and want of expression, seldom seen to the same degree in the drawings of primitive adults. The feature of distinction is above all the capacity for naturalistic reproduction of the outline, and particularly of motion. This is not only true of somewhat more advanced folk-art, but also of those of its products which are very primitive and nearest to the child's drawing.

[1] Hanna Rydh, *loc. cit.*, pp. 66, 67.

[2] E. R. Jaensch, *Über den Aufbau der Wahrnehmungswelt*, pp. 221 *et seq.*, 241, 242.

In Fig. 138, the human figures are formalized.   Arms
and legs are but simple lines, three dots show eyes and
mouth, and just as in the case of early children's
drawings, the nose is missing, but nevertheless the representation of the situation and action is full of life and
movement ; one person is lying stretched out on the
ground, another has just collapsed there, whilst two
others are still in fighting and defensive positions.   The
animal drawing in this case, as usually in primitive folk-
art, is better than the human figure.   Other parallels

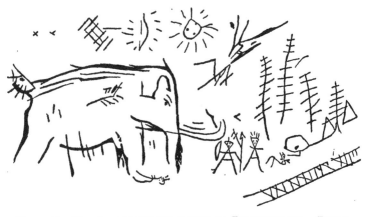

FIG. 138.—THE LENAPE STONE, FOUND IN PENNSYLVANIA.   REPRE-
SENTATION OF A MAMMOTH OR A MASTODON AND HUMAN BEINGS.
ABOUT 5/9. (FROM WILSON.)

to children's drawing are seen in the sun with a face
drawn in it, and the trees in feather formula.
     Even in drawings, made by older and gifted children,
which may be quite as true to nature as good folk-art,
there is generally something in the choice of the motive
or in the execution which enables us to guess the product
to be that of a child in civilized surroundings and not a
primitive savage.   A possibility of a mistake may exist
when older and talented children treat objects closely
connected with the life of primitive people, as in the case
of Levinstein's drawing by a fourteen-year-old boy of

Negro towns and an Indian camp.[1] Another example is a picture of trench warfare made by a ten-year-old boy, concerning which Hartlaub says quite rightly that it reminds us of drawings of the Stone Age and the Bushmen.[2]

Hartlaub also deals with the parallel problem. He thinks that only particularly gifted children can reveal what exists in every child. "Our reproductions show that four-year-old children, given water-colours and brush in place of a lead pencil, are able to produce pictures which are almost purely optical. Among the many drawings which then follow up to the eleventh year of age, some show the most astonishing similarity to cave drawings of the Diluvial Age, and those of the Bushmen." Hartlaub admits that the formula always precedes naturalistic representation in children's drawing ; but he points out that it is impossible to deny the assumption that naturalistic palæolithic art may have passed through a period of scribble and formula, even if we can find no traces of it. He therefore adheres to the validity of the biogenetic law in the matter of drawing although not to the chronological sequence which it gives.[3]

It is easy to understand that the astonishingly beautiful and naturalistic animal pictures from the best period of palæolithic art have attracted the attention of investigators to a high degree. It is not, however, correct that no traces of a period of scribbling and formula are to be found. After investigating as exactly as possible all material from palæolithic art available to me, I have arrived at the conclusion that we can find both scribbling and formula in the oldest period of palæolithic art, the Aurignac, and also many formalized features in later periods.

As a proof I reproduce here, alongside one another, a child's scribbled drawings of human heads with indications of body lines (Fig. 23) and the scribbled drawing

[1] Levinstein, loc. cit., p. 155, Plates 52, 53.
[2] Hartlaub, loc. cit., pp. 100, 161.　　[3] loc. cit., pp. 57, 58.

of a Stone Age man of animal heads with lines indicating
the body (Fig. 139).   The only difference between them
is, as usual, that the child draws human beings, the
Stone Age artist animals.   But otherwise both drawings
have exactly the same character.   In both the heads
are the best executed, the body lines are only indicated
incompletely ; in both, figures are placed one over the

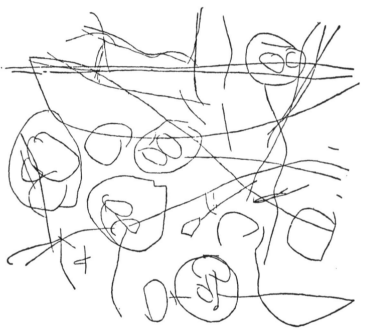

FIG. 23.—SCRIBBLE OF HUMAN HEADS WITH INDICATIONS OF BODY
    LINES. FROM MARGARET'S DRAWING FRAGMENT. 2 ; 7, 20.
    ABOUT 2/3.

other, and woven together in a tangle of lines going in
all directions without any definite orientation.
    Capitan and Peyrony assert that we may see in such
a Stone Age drawing of the Aurignac period the very
beginning of all art.   This beginning is the same in the
childhood of man as in that of mankind.   These investigators also point out that the indefinite and tangled

character of the drawings agrees with the mental life of Aurignac man, which was probably but little differentiated.[1]

The second example, also from the Aurignac period, is a rhinoceros, engraved on a stone tablet. Here again we have the impression of scribbled practice of the animal form ; figures cover one another to some extent, have no definite orientation, and are incompletely

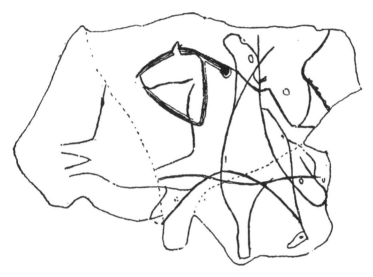

FIG. 139.—ENGRAVING OF ANIMAL HEADS WITH INDICATION OF BODY LINES. FROM THE OLDEST PALÆOLITHIC ART OF THE AURIGNAC PERIOD. (FROM CAPITAN AND PEYRONY.)

executed. Notice also some lines which have nothing to do with the figure, and are like the child's wavy scribble, as it would look if cut in stone instead of scribbled with pencil (Fig. 140).[2]

Cartailhac and Breuil report " an obvious scribble " (*véritable gribouillage*) from the Aurignac period in the

[1] Capitan et Peyrony, " Les origines de l'art à l'aurignacien moyen ", *Revue anthropologique*, 31, pp. 99, 100.
[2] Capitan, Breuil, Peyrony. Reproduced from Hanna Rydh, *loc. cit.*, p. 102.

Gargas Cave. On the walls or the roof a large number of tangled lines are engraved, and amongst this scribble we see primitive and more or less incomplete drawings of animals, horses, bison, and an elephant. In one place the soft clay of the cave roof has a tangle of lines drawn with the fingers, forming quite arbitrary and irregular loops and figures. Between these are animal forms, extraordinarily roughly executed and limited to the most elementary lines, but still such that one can clearly recognize the nature of the animal.[1]

In the cave of Hornos de la Pena similar scribbles of the earliest palæolithic period are to be found (Fig. 141).[2]

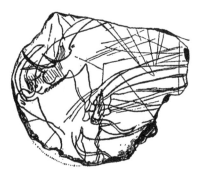

FIG. 140.—RHINOCEROS ENGRAVED ON A STONE SLAB IN THE TRILOBITE CAVE AT ARCY-SUR-CURE, YONNE. (FROM CAPITAN, BREUIL, AND PEYRONY.) REPRODUCED FROM HANNA RYDH.

Breuil found the same scribble mixed with primitive animal drawings in Altamira. As an example we give here a fragment showing, at the extreme left, a horse set vertically, with the want of definite orientation already referred to, and then a few lines which the authors interpret as an animal head with eyes, ears, and a portion of the line of the back ; at the top right a horse with the line of the back indicated, a *tétard* of the animal world ; below this a few scribbled lines which are supposed to

---

[1] Cartailhac et Breuil, " Les peintures et gravures murales des cavernes pyrénéennes ", *L'anthropologie*, 21, 1910, pp. 137 *et seq.*
[2] *loc. cit.*, p. 143.

have been made with a kind of tool having three grooves (Fig. 142).[1]

Scribble and rudimentary animal figures, mostly horses, drawn in a formalized and incomplete manner, have also been found in other caves. Details such as eyes, ears and feet are often missing, and sometimes even the legs. All of this is supposed by authorities to date from the beginning of the Aurignac period.[2]

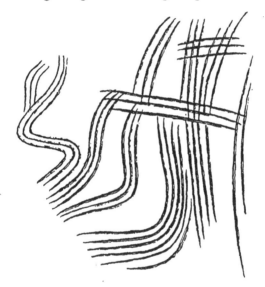

FIG. 141.—SCRIBBLE ON WALL OF THE CAVE HORNOS DE LA PENA. OLD STONE AGE. (FROM CARTAILHAC AND BREUIL.)

A similar mixture of scribble and more or less incomplete and formalized figures is also found, as we have seen, in children's drawing. A striking similarity is shown, for example, by Margaret's drawing at 1 ; 10, 5, which at the top right hand shows scribbling practice of straight lines and angles, and at the bottom on the left a formalized human figure (cf. p. 13). In this period of her drawing incomplete and formalized figures usually

[1] Cartailhac et Breuil, *loc. cit.*, pp. 144 *et seq.*   [2] *loc. cit.*, pp. 147, 148.

appeared in her scribblings, for example a flag-like shape, the outline of a flower, or a human formula. In the cave Pair-non-Pair there are a number of animal drawings of the Aurignac period carried out in so formalized and undifferentiated a fashion, that it is not even possible to determine the species of animal with certainty. They thus exhibit parallels with the formalized and undifferentiated animal drawings of children (Fig. 143).[1]

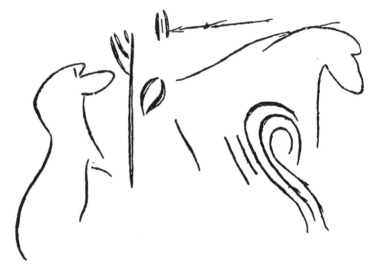

FIG. 142.—SCRIBBLE AND FORMALIZED ENGRAVINGS OF HORSES IN THE CAVE ALTAMIRA. OLD STONE AGE. AURIGNAC PERIOD. (FROM CARTAILHAC AND BREUIL.)

H. Shetelig reports that one often comes across incompletely executed representations of animals, drawn without plan over and between one another, in the rock engravings of the Norwegian Stone Age, and that we see, along with animal pictures, line forms, such as zig-zags, rectangles, triangles and irregular groups of lines. An example are the drawings on rock at Hell in

[1] Breuil et Cartailhac, " La caverne d'Altamira à Santillane (Espagne) ", 1906, p. 19, Fig. 8. (From Hanna Rydh, *loc. cit.*, p. 130.)

Stjördalen.[1] Some of them consist, according to G. Hallström, in a " chaotic tangle of strokes ", " an extraordinary mixture of ornament and body lines ".[2]

The cave art of southern countries exhibits similar simple geometrical lines and forms, " signs ", which have been named according to their supposed meaning : "house signs ", a rectangle divided by lines, " water sign ", parallel zig-zag lines, and so on. These belong to various periods (Fig. 144). They show great similarity to the child's practice scribble, zig-zag lines, wavy lines, rectangles, circles and so forth. Menghin also supposes that a great deal of this is only scribble.[3] But they

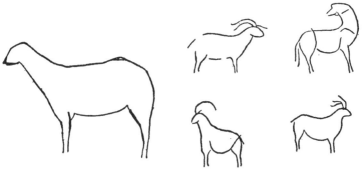

FIG. 143.—FORMALIZED ANIMAL DRAWINGS. ENGRAVINGS FROM THE CAVE PAIR-NON-PAIR, GIRONDE. (FROM CARTAILHAC AND BREUIL.) REPRODUCED FROM HANNA RYDH.

have also been interpreted, in common with the whole of palæolithic art, as the ritual expression of a magical activity already become complex. This view is founded on a comparison with other primitive races, including some at the present day, whose life is interwoven and directed by magical ideas and customs.[4]

[1] Shetelig, *Norges forhistorie*, pp. 39, 43.
[2] G. Hallström, "Hällristningar i norra Skandinavien ", *Ymer*, 1907, 221, 222. Hallström, "Nordskandinaviska Hällristningar ", *Fornvännen*, 1908, pp. 56 *et seq*.
[3] Hoernes-Menghin, *loc. cit.*, p. 675.
[4] L. Capitan, "Les manifestations ethnographiques et magiques sur les parois de la grotte de Montespan ", *Revue Anthropologique*, 33, pp. 545 *et seq*., 1923. *Cf.* Lévy-Bruhl, *La mentalité primitive*.

Regarded from the psychological point of view this conception appears to be built somewhat onesidedly upon the results of ethnology and race psychology. In the light of individual psychology, palæolithic art offers so many points of similarity with children's drawings, that it would appear more natural to regard it as the direct expression of the natural human tendency to representation, of an inborn sense for line and colour, in other

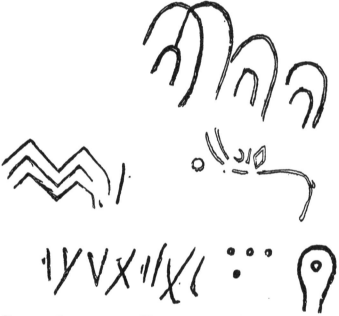

FIG. 144.—SIGNS FROM THE WALL OF THE CAVE MONTESPAN. (FROM CAPITAN.)

words, as an art for art's sake. Prehistorians such as Hoernes also put forward this view, at least as regards animal pictures.[1]

Luquet has already drawn attention to the onesidedness of the dominant psychological view of the artistic activity of Stone Age man. He has proved that the magical interpretation appears erroneous in at least

[1] Hoernes-Menghin, *loc. cit.*, pp. 185 *et seq.*

one respect. The pictures of human beings found in
the caves often have animal faces and animal-like figures ;
the arms are stretched forward and upwards, and the
legs are often sloping forwards or even almost horizontal.
The prehistorians have regarded them as " animal mask
dancers ", who are carrying out ritual ceremonies. The

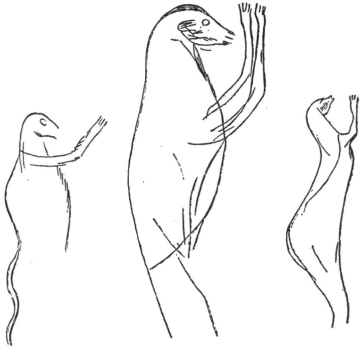

FIG. 145.—HUMAN FIGURES (SO-CALLED ANIMAL MASK DANCERS) FROM
THE CAVE ALTAMIRA. (FROM CARTAILHAC AND BREUIL.) REPRO-
DUCED FROM HANNA RYDH.

position of the legs is supposed to be an attempt to
represent dance movement, and the arms stretched upwards to express adoration (Fig. 145).[1]

Luquet shows that all the peculiar features of these

[1] Hanna Rydh, *loc. cit.*, pp. 149, 150. G. H. Luquet, " Sur les
caractères des figures humaines dans l'art paléolithique ", *L'Anthropologie*, 21, pp. 409 *et seq.* Concerning Mask Dances, see E. Grosse,
Die Anfänge der Kunst, pp. 181 *et seq.*

drawings of human figures are explained quite naturally by assuming that palæolithic artists, who drew animals almost exclusively, could not escape from animal form when they attempted to represent human beings. Their human beings are more or less vertical animal forms, just as the animal drawings of a child are human figures in a horizontal position (Fig. 146).[1] The Stone Age artist passed from the animal to the human being, just as the child passes from the human being to the animal, and both have the same primitive inability to master

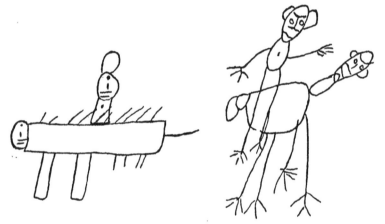

FIG. 146.—MAN AND HORSE. FORMALIZED DRAWINGS BY AN EIGHT-YEAR-OLD GIRL AND A SEVEN-YEAR-OLD BOY. (FROM KERS-CHENSTEINER.)

the unaccustomed form. Hoernes also gives it as his belief that the palæolithic artist was so accustomed to the animal form that his hand could only be brought with the greatest difficulty to carry out other lines. The " animal mask " from Trois Frères and a few other figures may perhaps be regarded as exceptions, although there can be no objection to regarding them in the same way.[2]

The fact that palæolithic artists prefer to represent

[1] Luquet, *loc. cit.*, pp. 409 *et seq.*
[2] Hoernes-Menghin, *loc. cit.*, pp. 170, 668 *et seq.*

animals has also been interpreted in the magical sense. It is supposed to indicate a supplication to unknown powers for rich booty in the hunt, or a kind of charm to bring the animals into the power of the hunter.[1] But the persistent choice of the animal motive may also be explained purely psychologically. A hunter with a taste for art will naturally try to represent, above all things, the animals which he hunts, for his whole thought and action are devoted to overcoming them, and their lines and forms are engraved on his memory, after a hard day's hunting, with almost hallucinatory clearness.[2] When the animals are represented from the side as wounded by spear or arrow, a confirmation of the magical interpretation has been found in this fact.[3] This is supposed to cry aloud the meaning of the work of art.[4] But here also the magical interpretation is not indispensable ; for the fact is psychologically just as natural as when a child seldom draws a horse by itself, but usually adds a cart or a rider on its back. If we do not see the hunter who has shot the arrow as well, the cause may be sought in want of power to represent the human figure.

Luquet, in a paper on realism in palæolithic art, has shown that several formalized characteristics exist which are found again in all periods, even in the latest Madeleine period, and are paralleled in children's drawing. Things of lesser interest are left out, such as the eyes, ears and arms of the human figure ; the point of an arrow is always drawn, but the shaft is often omitted. The object is shown simultaneously from every point of view usually in its " orthoscopic form "—the animal in profile has its form drawn full face, the feet seen from above, and so on. Cases of transparency are also not wanting—the arrow-head, although sticking in the animal's body, is visible ; internal organs such as the alimentary

---

[1] A. W. Brögger, " Billedkunst og magi ", _Det norske folk i oldtiden_, pp. 72 _et seq._
[2] Hoernes-Menghin, _loc. cit._, pp. 13, 14, 125, 126.
[3] Paulsen, _Urtidens kunst_, p. 53.
[4] Hanna Rydh, _loc. cit._, pp. 76 _et seq._, 174.

canal, the heart, or the skeleton are indicated. Luquet therefore maintains that palæolithic art, up to well in the Madeleine period, shows an æsthetic which is in many respects similar to that of the child.[1]

Common features are also found in the continual repetition of the same object, and in the decided want of synthesis—various animals are represented singly, and one only finds here and there attempts at a composition—and further in the want of spatial arrangement, in indifferent orientation or even spatial displacement, further also in the defective power of representing more rapid movement. The animals are mostly represented standing, lying down, or moving slowly.[2]

The most ancient folk-art therefore begins, like that of the child, with scribbling and formalized drawing, both of which play the same part as in children's drawing. Lines and forms are played with, strokes and figures are practised by scribbling, and these are later used to carry out complete drawings. Palæolithic art gradually develops from scribbling and formula until it reaches its highest point in the beautiful naturalistic polychrome paintings of the Madeleine period (Fig. 147). There can be no question that its development is a parallel to the development of children's drawing, such as we see in the typical series of Margaret's drawing which have been given as examples ; these also show the development from scribbling and formula to many coloured, comparatively naturalistic drawings.[3] That palæolithic art

[1] G. H. Luquet, " Le réalisme dans l'art paléolithique ", L'Anthropologie, 33, pp. 17 et seq., 1923.
[2] For this comparison I have paid particular attention to French and North Spanish Cave Art, as being the best known. The East Spanish has a somewhat different character, but develops parallel with the first named, according to Obermaier (loc. cit., p. 189).
[3] I assume that the statements made by first-class French investigators concerning the chronological development of palæolithic art are correct. Obermaier cites them, following H. Breuil in the Prähistorische Zeitschrift, 13/14, pp. 183/84, 1921/22. Hence I take no account of the criticism of Hoernes and Menghin concerning the comparison between children's drawing and folk-art, as their criticism is based on the view that no progressive development can be shown to exist in palæolithic art.

was more naturalistic from the beginning than children's drawing has nothing to do with the fact of this parallelism.

The comparison between children's drawing and palæolithic thus confirms the biogenetic law that the development of the species is reproduced in the child. But if all races and periods are taken into account, there can be no question of a simple and exact agreement, of a repetition in chronological succession, but at the very most, recapitulation with many gaps, overlappings, and displacements. One could only expect a more complete parallelism to appear in continuous periods of development. Lamprecht's proposal to historicize the ethnographical facts by means of children's drawings would therefore be erroneous.

As Claparède has pointed out, the parallelism expressed in the biogenetic law can also be explained by the fact that nature always makes use of the same means to further the development of the individual as well as that of the species.[1] Parallels in the manifestation of the psychical life, in speech, drawing, and so on, may also be explained in a third manner. This reason for parallelism is to be found in the like character of the primitive and undeveloped mental life of both child and primitive man ; in comparing children's drawing with primitive folk-art in general, this last explanation is probably the best founded.

The unquestioned parallels, which can be shown between the drawing of primitive man and that of children—formalism, transparency, turning-over, spacelessness, want of synthesis—are based on features common to the psyche of the child and primitive man, on the want of firm voluntary attention, of penetrating analysis and higher synthesis, on the weakness of the power of abstraction and of logical and realistic thinking.[2] When we find these features of children's drawings repeated

[1] E. Claparède, *Psychologie de l'enfant*. 9th Ed. Geneva, 1922, p. 531. [2] *Cf.* Lévy-Bruhl, *La mentalité primitive*.

again in primitive art, we may conclude that their executants were similar in their psychical make-up. Rouma therefore goes too far in maintaining that no conclusions can be drawn from a comparison.

Along with the many points of similarity there are also many differences. A number of these differences must be referred to the gap which always exists between children and adults, in spite of common features of primitive development. The adult is riper; the drawing of the child is play, that of the adult art; the adult has more power of observation, more mental pictures, greater skill of hand. Other differences are conditioned by environment, occupation, religion, thought, social conditions, so that the difference between the art of the Stone Age and the drawing of gifted civilized children may be explained. Similar causes are also partly at the bottom of the great differences found between the art of individual primitive peoples, thus, for example, that between the art of the Old Stone Age and the following periods, between that of the Bushmen and the Bantu. If to this is added a difference in inherited artistic capacity and artistic tradition we have an explanation why peoples living otherwise under approximately similar conditions, such as hunters with sharp powers of observation and great skill of hand, none the less follow greatly different paths in the matter of artistic production.

Even if we are not able to determine the level of culture of a race from its art without further question, we may none the less draw conclusions from pictorial art concerning many characteristics of the psychical and cultured development of a race. The study of children's drawing may assist us to a correct interpretation, since it gives a generally valid expression for important features in the general development of human mentality.

BIBLIOGRAPHY

J. M. Baldwin, *Die Entwicklung des Geistes beim Kinde und bei der Rasse*, Berlin, 1898.

Earl Barnes, " A Study of Children's Drawings ". *PdSe*, 2, pp. 455–463, 1892. *Studies in Education*, 1, 2nd edn., 1903 ; 2, 1902.

W. Bechterew, " Recherches objectives sur l'évolution du dessin chez l'enfant ". *JPsNa*, 1911, IX, X.

L. Belinfante-Ahn, *Het Kinderteekenen en het volle Leven*, Zeist, 1920.

O. Bic, " Zur Entwicklung des Auges ", *Kind und Kunst*, 1905, II., pp. 157–159.

F. Breest, " Ein kleiner Künstler ", *Kind und Kunst*, 1905, VIII., pp. 333–335.

Elmer E. Brown, " Notes on Children's Drawings." *University of California Publications in Education*, 2 (1), 1897.

K. Bühler, *The Mental Development of the Child*, London, 1933.

A. H. Chamberlain, *The Child*, London, 3rd edn., 1900.

E. Cirese, " T disegni infantile ", *RPs(i)*, 5 (3), pp. 248–254, 1909.

E. Claparède, " Plan d'expériences collectives sur le dessin des enfants ", *ArPs(f)*, 6 Jan., 1907, pp. 276–278.

A. Clark, " The Children's Attitude toward Perspective Problems ", *SdEd*, 1, pp. 283–294.

E. Cooke, *The ABC of Drawing*, Special Reports on Educational Subjects, 1896–97, Educational Dpt., London. pp. 115 *et seq.*, 1897.

Louisa McDermott, " Favourite Drawings of Indian Children ", *North Western Monthly*, 8, pp. 134–137, 1897.

Alice Descoedres, *Le développement de l'enfant de deux à sept ans*. Neuchatel and Paris, 1921.

" Couleur, forme, ou nombre ", *ArPs(f)*, 14 (16), 1914 ; 16 (61), 1916.

Deutsche Kunsterziehung, L. Pallat, G. Kerschensteiner, and others. Berlin and Leipzig, 1908.

K. W. Dix, *Körperliche und geistige Entwicklung eines Kindes*. 2. *Die Sinne*. Leipzig, 1912, pp. 67 *et seq.*

J. Dück, " Über das zeichnerische und künstlerische Interesse der Schüler ", *ZPdPs*, 13, pp. 172–177, 1912.

Helga Eng, *Kunstpädagogik*, Oslo, 1918.

Margaret Gallagher, " Children's Spontaneous Drawings ", *North Western Monthly*, 8, pp. 130–134, 1897.

C. Götze, *Das Kind als Künstler*, Hamburg, 1898.

Florence L. Goodenough, *The Measurement of Intelligence by Drawings*, New York, 1926.

H. Grosser and W. Stern, *Das freie Zeichnen und Formen des Kindes*. Collection of papers from *ZAngPs*. Leipzig, 1913.

G. F. Hartlaub, *Das Genius im Kinde*, Breslau, 1922.

Louise Hogan, *A Study of a Child*, New York, 1898.

E. Ivanoff, *Récherchés expérimentales sur le dessin des écoliers de la Suisse romande*, Geneva, 1908.

E. R. Jaensch, *Über den Aufbau der Wahrnehmungswelt und ihre Struktur im Jugendalter*, Leipzig, 1923.

M. D. Katzaroff, " Q'est-ce que les enfants dessinent ? " *ArPs(f)*, 9, pp. 125–133, 1910.

D. Katz, " Ein Beitrag zur Kenntnis der Kinderzeichnungen ", *Zeitschrift für Psychologie*, 41, pp. 241–256, 1906.

G. Kerschensteiner, *Die Entwicklung der zeichnerischen Begabung*, Munich, 1905.

C. Kik, " Die übernormale Zeichenbegabung bei Kindern ", *ZAngPs*, 2, pp. 92–149, 1909.

P. Krause, *Entwicklung eines Kindes*, Leipzig, 1914.

J. Kretschmar, " Sammlungen freier Kinderzeichnungen ", *ZAngPs*, 3, pp. 459–463, 1918.
" Die freie Kinderzeichnung in der wissenschaftlichen Forschung ", *ZPdPs*, 13, pp. 380–394, 1912.

W. Krötzsch, *Rhythmus und Form in der freien Kinderzeichnung*, Leipzig, 1917.

S. Levinstein, *Kinderzeichnungen bis zum 14ten. Lebensjahr*, Leipzig, 1905.

M. Lobsien, " Kinderzeichnungen und Kunstkanon ", *ZPdPs*, 7, pp. 393–404, 1905.

H. Lukens, " A Study of Children's Drawings in the Early Years ", *PdSe*, 4, pp. 79–101, 1896.
" Die Entwicklungsstufen beim Zeichnen ", *Kinderfehler* (Langensalza), 2, pp. 166–177, 1897.

G.-H. Luquet, *Les dessins d'un enfant*, Paris, 1913.
" Le premier age du dessin enfantin ", *ArPs(f)*, 1912, II.
" Les bonhommes têtards dans le dessin enfantin ", *JPsNa*, 17, pp. 684–710, 1920.
Le dessin enfantin, Paris, 1927.

Louise Maitland, " What Children draw to please Themselves ", *Inland Educator*, Sept. 1st, 1895, pp. 77–81.
" Notes on Eskimo Drawings ", *North Western Monthly*, June 9th, 1899, pp. 443–450.

D. R. Major, *First Steps in Mental Growth*, New York, 1906.

W. Matz, " Zeichen und Modellierversuch an Volksschülern, Hilfsschülern, Taubstummen, und Blinden." *ZAngPs*, 10, pp. 52–135, 1915.

G. Fr. Muth, " Über Ornamentationsversuche mit Kindern im Alter von 6–9 Jahren ", *ZAngPs*, 6, pp. 21–50, 1913.

L. Nagy, *Fejezetek a gyermekrajzok lélektanából*, Budapesth, 1905.

Lena Partridge, " Children's Drawings of Men and Women ",
    SdEd, 2, pp. 163–179.
J. Passy, " Notes sur les dessins d'enfants ", *Revue Philosophique*,
    32, pp. 614–621, 1891.
G. Penazza, " La scrittura-disegno e il disegno-scrittura ", *RPs(i)*,
    4 (1), 1908.
B. Perez, *L'Education intellectuelle dès le berceau*, Paris, 1901 :
    Chap. X, " Le Dessin ", pp. 207–244.
L'Art et la poésie chez l'enfant, Paris, 1888.
R. Peter, " Beiträge zur Analyse der zeichnerischen Begabung ",
    ZPdPs, 15, pp. 96–104, 1914.
W. Pfleiderer, *Die Geburt des Bildes*, Stuttgart, 1930.
M. Probst, " Les dessins des enfants kabyles " *ArPs(f)*, 6,
    pp. 131–140, 1907.
Vilh. Rasmussen, *Børnehavebarnet. Verdensbillede og begavelse*,
    Copenhagen and Christiania, 1918.
C. Ricci, *L'arte dei bambini*, Bologna, 1887. Leipzig, 1906.
Anna M. Roos, " Barnet som konstnär ", *Ord. och Bilde*, 1908,
    pp. 337 *et seq.*
G. Rouma, *Le langage graphique de l'enfant*, Brussels, 2nd edn.,
    1913.
W. J. Ruttmann, *Die Ergebnisse der bisherigen Untersuchungen
    zur Psychologie des Zeichnens*, Leipzig, 1911.
M. C. Schuyten, " De oorspronkelijke ' Ventjes ' der Antwerpsche
    Schoolkindern ", *Paedologisch Jaarboek*, 5, 1904.
E. and G. Scupin, *Bubis erste Kindheit*, Leipzig, 1907.
Bubi im vierten bis sechsten Lebensjahre, Leipzig, 1910.
W. Stern, " Die zeichnerische Entwicklung eines Knaben vom 4.
    bis zum 7. Jahre ", *ZAngPs*, 3, pp. 1–31, 1910.
" Über verlagerte Raumformen ", *ZAngPs*, 2, pp. 498–526,
    1909.
Köhler, Verworn, Kretschmar, " Sammlungen freier Kinder-
    zeichnungen ", *ZAngPs*, 1, pp. 179, 472 ; 2, p. 180 ; 3,
    p. 459.
Psychologie der frühen Kindheit, Leipzig, 1914.
J. Sully, *Studies of Childhood*, London, 1896.
H. Volkelt, " Primitive Komplexqualitäten in Kinderzeich-
    nungen ", *Bericht über den VIII Kongress für experimentelle
    Psychologie in Leipzig*, Jena, 1914, pp. 204–208 ; *Fort-
    schritte der experimentellen Kinderpsychologie*, Jena, 1926.
O. Wulff, *Die Kunst des Kindes*, Stuttgart, 1927.

PREHISTORIC ART, ETC.

Bourlon, " Nouvelles decouvertes à Laugerie-Basse. Rabots, os
    utilités, oeuvres d'art ", *L'anthropologie*, 27, pp. 1–26, 1916.
H. Breuil, " Nouvelles figurations humaines de la caverne David
    à Cabrerets ", *RAnt*, 34, pp. 165–171, 1924.
" Les roches peintes de Minateda ", *L'anthropologie*, 30, pp.
    1–50, 1920.

L. Lévy-Bruhl, *La mentalité primitive*, Paris, 2nd edn., 1922.
Les fonctions mentales dans les sociétés inférieures, Paris, 5th edn., 1922.

A. W. Brøgger, " Det norske folk i oldtiden ", *Instituttet for sammenlignende kulturforskning*, Series A. 6a. Oslo, 1925.

L. Capitan, " Les manifestations ethnographiques et magiques sur les parois de la grotte de Montespan ", *RAnt*, 33, pp. 545 *et seq.*, 1923.

L. Capitan and D. Peyrony, " Les origines de l'art à l'aurignacien moyen ", *RAnt*, 31, pp. 92–112, 1921.

E. Cartailhac and H. Breuil, " Les peintures et gravures murales des cavernes pyrénéennes. IV. Gargas ". *L'anthropologie*, 21, pp. 129–150, 1910.

K. Doehlemann, " Prähistorische Kunst und Kinderzeichnungen ", *Beiträge zur Anthropologie und Urgeschichte*, 1908, p. 51.

A. van Gennep, " Dessins d'enfant et dessin préhistorique ", *ArPs(f)*, Feb. 10th, 1911, pp. 327–337.

E. Grosse, *Die Anfänge der Kunst,* Freiburg i. B., 1894.

G. Hallström, " Hällristningar i norra Skandinavien ", *Ymer*, 27, 1907, Stockholm, 1908, pp. 211–227.
" Nordskandinaviska hällristningar. II. De norska ristningarna ", *Fornvännen*, 2, 3, 4, 1907–1909.

Yrjø Hirn, *Konstens Ursprung*, Stockholm, 1902.

M. Hoernes-Menghin, *Urgeschichte der bildenden Kunst in Europa*, Vienna, 1925.

J. Kretschmar, " Kinderkunst und Urzeitkunst ", *ZPdPs*, 1910, pp. 354–366.

K. Lamprecht, " Les dessins d'enfant comme source historique ", *Bulletin de l'Académie royale de Belgique (classe des lettres, etc.)*, No. 9–10, pp. 457–469, 1906.
Appendix : In Levinstein, " Kinderzeichnungen ".

G.-H. Luquet, " Sur les caractères des figures humaines dans l'art paléolithique ", *L'anthropologie*, 21, pp. 409–423, 1910.
" Le réalisme dans l'art paléolithique ", *L'anthropologie*, 33, pp. 17–48, 1923.

G. Montandon, " Gravures et peintures rupestres des indiens du cataract Canyon Arizona ", *L'anthropologie*, 33, pp. 347–355, 1923.

H. Obermaier, " Paleolithikum und steinzeitliche Felskunst in Spanien. Übersichten ", *Prähistorische Zeitschrift*, 13–14, pp. 177–199, 1921–22.

F. Paulsen, " Urtidens Kunst ", *Kultur og videnskab.*, 5, Copenhagen, 1923.

Ed. Piette, " Les galets coloriés du Mas d'Azil ", supplement to No. 4, July–August, 1896, of the review *L'anthropologie*.

S. Reinach, *L'art quaternaire*, Paris, 1913.

F. Rosen, " Darstellende Kunst im Kindesalter der Völker ", *ZAngPs*, 1, pp. 93–118, 1907.

Hanna Rydh, *Grottmänniskornas årtusenden*, Stockholm, 1926.

H. Shetelig, *Norsk kunst i de eldste tider*. *Norsk kunsthistorie*, Oslo, 1925.

" Norges forhistorie. Problemer og resultater i norsk arkaeologie, *Instituttet for sammenlignende kulturforskning*, Series A. 5a. Oslo, 1925.

M. Verworn, " Zur Psychologie der primitiven Kunst ", *Naturwissenschaftliche Wochenschrift*, 22(46), 1907.

Ideoplastische Kunst, 1914.

" Kinderkunst und Urgeschichte ", *Korrespondenzblatt der deutschen Gesellschaft für Anthropologie*, 38, pp. 42–46, 1907.

T. Wilson, " The Prehistoric Art. Report of the U.S. National Museum ". *Annual Report of the Smithsonian Institution*, pp. 325–664, Washington, 1898.

W. Wundt, *Elemente der Völkerpsychologie*, Leipzig, 1912.

ABBREVIATIONS

ArPs(*f*) = *Archives de Psychologie*.
JPsNa = *Journal de Psychologie normale et pathologique*.
PdSe = *Pedagogical Seminary*.
RAnt = *Revue anthropologique des écoles d'anthropologie de Paris et de Liège*.
RPs(*i*) = *Rivista di Psicologia*.
SdEd = *Studies in Education*, Ed. by Earl Barnes, Philadelphia.
ZAngPs = *Zeitschrift für angewandte Psychologie*.
ZPdPs = *Zeitschrift für pädagogische Psychologie*.

INDEX

221